VICTORIOUS AGING

TIPS FOR YOUR BEST HEALTH AT ANY AGE

VICTORIOUS AGING

TIPS FOR YOUR BEST HEALTH AT ANY AGE

Dr. Martha Lucas, L.AC.

www.acupuncturewoman.com

ARMLIN HOUSE

ArmLin House Productions
P.O. Box 2522, Littleton, Colorado 80161-2522
www.armlinhouse.com

ISBN: 978-1-958185-39-1

Cover Design by Dancing Tornado Designs
www.dancingtornado.com

Printed in the United States of America

First Edition

CONTENTS

To my loving family—my husband, children, and grandchildren—whose unwavering support, encouragement, and laughter fill my life with purpose and joy.

And to my patients, past and present, who have trusted me with their stories, their healing, and their hopes.

You all inspire me daily and give me the space, strength, and spirit to write, teach, and do what I love.

This book is for you.

OBSESSION

CHAPTER 1

Aging is not lost youth but a new stage of
opportunity and strength.

> – Betty Friedan

OUR SOCIETY IS obsessed with how we look, especially with appearing young. We're bombarded with a crazy amount of safe and unsafe, as well as healthy and unhealthy, ways to change how we look to achieve the desired level of youthfulness. It's a modern fixation, this quest to look younger, live longer, and feel energetic. We desire fewer symptoms of aging, which is why a plethora of ads push us to spend money on diets, equipment, testing, procedures, and a wealth of ingenious new ways to fight off aging.

Anti-aging efforts, such as using natural skin care products and making healthy lifestyle choices, mitigate the visible signs of aging; however, achieving the flawless appearance seen in Photoshopped images is unrealistic. These images create the illusion of youth by erasing wrinkles, blemishes, and other natural features that come with age. Actual skin has texture and actual bodies change over time. Embracing natural changes, rather than striving for the impossible standard presented in Photoshopped images, promotes healthier self-esteem and well-being. While anti-aging products and routines enhance our appearance, they cannot and should not replace the authenticity of a life well-lived.

Consider cultures that accept aging and recognize it as a natural progression of life. In Eastern cultures, such as China and Japan, people revere aging and respect their elders for their wisdom and experience. Older generations often live with their extended families. Younger people are taught to honor and care for their elders. In African and Native American communities, they integrate aging into their social fabric. Elders are knowledge keepers and pillars of the community. Their contributions are deeply valued. But in the United States, aging is associated with a decline in productivity, and seniors live in retirement communities rather than with their families.

The emphasis on youth and beauty is nothing new, as well as being a very well-researched phenomenon. Here are a few of the questions the research has answered:

- **Why does beauty fade as we age?** Sun damage causes elastin in the skin to breakdown leading to wrinkles and sagging.

- **At what age do looks/beauty decline?** Women over the age of 40 start to decline and look older, while it's over 50 for men.

- **What face shape ages the slowest?** A round face with full cheeks and natural plumpness best maintains a youthful appearance.

It's unfortunate our society despises the effects of aging. We perceive almost everything associated with aging as unwanted and ugly. Hence, the thriving multi-billion-dollar market of products and services for erasing the effects of aging.

The Grandparent Effect

Our expectations affect our behavior (self-fulfilling prophecy) and other's behavior toward us. Consider being a grandparent. For centuries, in many cultures, elders have played a critical role in sharing wisdom and providing social and economic support to their families and kinship groups. Today, people routinely live long enough to become grandparents and great grandparents. But if being called "Grandma" is a negative label, and if it implies that we're elderly, then we may feel older and that may lead others to treat us as if we're older.

The culture of grandparents and ageism is interesting. According to research, an involved grandparent is associated with improved health and well-being. Yet many grandparents, me included, are occasionally asked if being a grandparent makes them feel old. No, it doesn't make me feel old; it makes me feel young. A lot of grandparents don't see themselves as aging, they see themselves as young. Grandchildren take us back to our younger days: running in the park, playing on the floor with blocks, swinging on a swing set, romping on the splash pad at the lake, or sliding at the water park. We bake cookies, play in the snow, and laugh a lot. None of this makes me feel old. Being a grandparent adds a layer of meaningfulness to one's life instead of being an "I'm old now" curse. It's an anti-aging factor for many grandparents. It helps them feel the *rapture of being alive*: the only purpose in life according to author Joseph Campbell.

What Is Anti-Aging Anyway?

We can't stop the clock! Wouldn't it make more sense to be obsessed with feeling good, living healthy, and accepting ourselves with what I call "victorious aging?" Because guess what? Aging does not equal decaying. We can change our game and continue healthy development. Yes, let's reframe aging as development. It's another stage in the development of life. I don't run a 7-minute mile like my grandson or 9.5-minute mile like my daughter does, but I *can* and *do* run. It's the same idea as shifting gears when you mountain bike. You don't pedal the entire ride in one gear. Frankly, that would be stupid. The same thing with your car. Changing gears is normal. It's natural. It's expected and accepted. It's the same with *aging well*–or rather *developing well* in our later years. As we age, we can take charge of change by incorporating exercise, healthy food, a positive attitude, meditation, chanting, and self-love into our lives. As a result, we become better, stronger, and faster, even when we already feel our healthiest because that's the only way we'll ever know how healthy we can be! It's about believing in what's possible rather than accepting what others say is impossible. When my oldest grandson turned 17, my response was, "Wow! I don't *feel* 17 years older." In fact, I felt better than ever. Interesting because I am indeed 17 years older.

Part of an anti-aging lifestyle may indeed include interventions more "dramatic" than natural skin care, exercise, healthy diet, etc. Perhaps you have arthritis in your knees but want to continue your athletic activities. You may opt for a cortisone injection in your knee so you can stay active. Exercise is very important for successful aging–physically *and* emotionally. Injections are a choice you would make to maintain the same level of activity. You may say, 'Dr. Martha, I can't believe you said getting a cortisone injection is okay.' Look at it this way: arthritis is going to continue to progress with or without the injections. Sure, you can quit running or stop activities that keep you healthy, but arthritis will still progress. Arthritis will win.

Don't get me wrong; I want to look young and vibrant as well as remain as healthy as possible while I age. There's no doubt that maintaining a healthy, younger look takes *lifestyle actions*, not just procedures. There isn't one procedure that will do it for you. It's your lifestyle that will do it for you. Just sitting back and allowing the clock to tick results in looking older, especially if you avoid efforts to take care of your health.

Aging Is Not Decaying

Aging isn't decaying. It's a process. Consider your aging car. When your brake pads are old and worn, they squeak when you brake. What do you do when this happens? Either you repair them or let the situation get worse. It's the same with your health. When you identify issues that interfere with your well-being (i.e., changes in your hair, skin, posture, digestion, or overall health), you intervene and see a specialist, or you wait for the symptoms to worsen and become more difficult to resolve.

We *know* when our body changes. Unfortunately, people wrongly believe that aging means waiting for the body to fall apart. *Not true!* Aging does not need to include these things:

- **Depression and loneliness**. Studies show that older adults are less likely to experience depression than their younger counterparts.

- **Less sleep**. Older adults still need 7 to 9 hours of sleep a night. Sleep is very important for good health.

- **Lack of learning and dementia**. Older adults can learn things and improve skills. In fact, learning something new improves overall memory. Dementia is not a normal part of aging.

When we consider our health and well-being a development, a project, a choice to age well, it is easier to think of aging as a continuous journey. Taking care of your health along the way is far better than recovering from illness and disability. It *is* possible to avoid illness and live healthily.

When we are healthy, when we feel healthy, improved appearance follows. Your skin is bright, your eyes are shiny, your body is fit. Aging doesn't take a huge toll when you maintain good health rather than searching for procedures to make you look younger or help you feel better. Over time, our bodies change, and possibilities present themselves. Do we need to pay attention to these changes? Yes.

Why Am I So Passionate About Aging?

I have been interested in the topic of beauty for many years, even before I began my career in Traditional Chinese Medicine (TCM). I worked as a Research Psychologist and studied issues in social and health psychology. As a researcher, I focused on what I could see, feel, weigh, and measure. That's what researchers do: observe and measure. One of my research areas was the study of attractiveness. Research shows that perceived attractiveness leads to positive outcomes: the more captivating others perceive a person, the more likely he, she, or they are to get the job, find a mate, and be considered as more intelligent. This is referred to as the "attractiveness halo effects" because positive attributes like intelligence, timeliness, honesty, etc. are attributed to people perceived as "attractive." Regardless of your IQ, if you're beautiful, people think you are smart. This explains why money follows our obsession with attractiveness. Americans spend billions of dollars on cosmetic procedures that promise to remove wrinkles, enhance skin, plump lips, full cheeks, lift eyelids, tuck bellies, and more.

I have been a practitioner of TCM for over twenty years and have seen how prevention, self-care, and natural remedies can slow down or nearly negate some results of aging. Plus, when we use natural medicine to stay healthy, if or when we become ill or require a medical procedure, we are more likely to rapidly heal and combat aging effects. For example, my patients who receive regular acupuncture treatments are sick less frequently. If they catch a cold or the flu, it goes away quickly. Often, there is no need for doctor visits or meds like antibiotics. Those who receive regular acupuncture and experience a stressful event have less gray hair than other non-treated people. I know from personal experience that highly stressful situations—a child almost dying—are easier on the mind, body, and soul when you have been taking care of yourself.

Acupuncture trains the body to be healthier and respond more quickly and efficiently to stressors. But let's say you don't have access to acupuncture. There are herbal formulae options, what I refer to as "acupuncture treatment in between acupuncture treatment." Chinese herbal prescriptions energetically affect the body similarly to acupuncture. Bottom line, I create plans that support existing health and encourage positive aging.

The search for youth, vitality, and beauty seems endless. And so is the list of procedures we have been willing to endure to achieve this goal, including suctioning, injections, chemical peels, implants, dyes & spray tans, cosmetic surgery, and the list goes on ...

As a specialist in Cosmetic Acupuncture, I'm amazed by the procedures that people willingly undergo when the technique promises a younger or more beautiful look, no matter what the negative side effects. And I'm frustrated that people have natural options such as Cosmetic Acupuncture that really works. Unfortunately, people choose more aggressive and dangerous options that can lead to harmful outcomes, even when there are no guarantees of perfect results. But first, let's take a moment to look inside you.

Reflective Questions

Read the following questions and take a moment to think about each. Then grab a notebook and write down your well thought out answers.

1. Do you like the way you look? Do you like what you see when you look in the mirror?

2. When you look in the mirror, are there things about your face you dislike or wish to change?

3. How do you feel about your body? Are you unhappy with your weight?

4. Have you searched for ways to minimize smile lines on your face?

5. Are you prematurely gray or despise your gray, silver, or white hair?

6. Do you wake up feeling energetic and well rested?

7. How often do you need to take time off work or other activities because of illness?

8. Do you recover quickly from injuries and illnesses?

9. When was the last time that you relaxed with a facial mask–such as a moisturizing clay mask–as self-care?

Satisfaction Not Guaranteed

I rarely hear how satisfied people are with their appearance and health. Usually, it's the opposite. There's always a wrinkle here, a wrinkle there, more than one chin, puffiness under the eyes, age spots, belly fat, lethargy, and a slew of other problems to talk about. That's why, when women consult with me about Cosmetic Acupuncture, I always ask what they like about their face. I then remind them that our faces are the result of heredity and life experience (excessive smiling), and that we want to *enhance* the results of our life experiences, not *erase* them.

Who are we comparing ourselves to, anyway? Women on the covers of fashion magazines? Well, we will never measure up to those images because that's what they are: Photoshopped images. I suppose with enough surgery, plumping injections, implants, liposuction, permanent makeup, and airbrushing, maybe, just maybe, we could look something like those women on magazine covers. But it's unlikely, and how would we maintain it? Society's messages are hard to accept:

Youth = Beauty
Youth = Perfection
Youth = Flawless

If you must undergo surgery to achieve a certain look, is it worth it? The idea that beauty is flawless and youthful is just not true. I have many female patients in their 70s, 80s, and 90s, and they are beautiful!

One patient, who I'll call Noreen, would arrive to clinic all dressed up during the holidays. She would wear a sequin dress, have her hair pulled up in a fancy bun, and dance the light fantastic on her way into the clinic. I'd think how I wanted to have that much energy and verve when I'm 86.

Then there's Samantha, a 92-year-old who I also find beautiful. She has a heart so big that she makes it her mission to improve other's lives, including adding healthier choices to the cafeteria menu at the assisted living facility where she lives. She read my book, *Catholic Daughters of Catholic Mothers: A Memoir and Guided Journal* and it inspired her to write her memoir to share her secrets of feeling fulfilled through life's little challenges.

And last but not least, there's Lynne, who always wears a "Life is Good" t-shirt when she visits me. At 84 years young, she left an unhappy marriage to go out on her own, with some help from family, and has her own happy place now. These are what I call beautiful and ageless women!

Another very serious issue is that it's not even older women who seek invasive procedures. Women in their twenties are already unhappy with their looks and try to measure up to societal images by undergoing procedures. Even some teenagers desire procedures like breast augmentation to feel better about their bodies. If we start sharing a healthier attitude about our bodies and faces around young women, they won't pursue plastic surgery when they're young.

Anti-Aging Obsession and Chinese Medicine

I am blessed to know, use, and teach TCM, a healthy way of minimizing the effects of aging. TCM includes safe treatments and a commitment to lifestyle changes anyone can follow. And that's what this book will address: ways to find your healthy, anti-aging plan. I am optimistic that TCM can end the boundless searches for unhealthy or even dangerous procedures we hope will fulfill our vanity needs.

Although obsessing over how one looks and feels may start at an early age, it's more clearly an issue when women reach our 40s and begin perimenopause. TCM calls this stage of a woman's life our "second spring." We now have the freedom to nourish ourselves and regenerate. Our focus changes from caring for young children to caring for ourselves and pursuing interests we didn't have time for earlier in our lives. It's a time to replenish our stores of energy for our future. According to Chinese medicine, we enter a liberating phase of life.

It's important to approach perimenopause changes with self-compassion. In Chinese medicine, these changes are viewed more positively compared to other cultures. I encourage women to think about perimenopause as a developmental stage of life—a renovation, just like having a monthly period used to be. Acceptance and willingness to make a few changes can make the journey through our "second spring" a success.

This book will help you discover how to redefine the limits of aging well. I will provide information, explanations, and alternatives to help change your bad habits and create positive ones. And you'll create your own anti-aging plan by completing the questionnaire at the end of each chapter. Now let's start by finding out how you feel about aging and your specific desires for aging well.

Your Anti-Aging Checklists

How Do You Feel About Aging?

Here you will answer questions about how you feel about aging and how it fits into your lifestyle.

1. What's your cultural experience with aging?

2. Every year, on your birthday, do you expect to feel older?

3. Imagine you don't know your age and must guess. How old do you feel?

4. Have you seen the movie *Lost Horizon?* The main guru says that knowing our age makes us live shorter lives. Do you think that knowing your age limits you from doing things you believe are only for younger people?

5. What are your personal expectations about aging?

6. What do you want for your health as you age?

7. Are you a grandparent? If so, how does it make you feel about your age?

8. Do you maintain your body's health like you maintain your car's health?

9. How does looking in the mirror make you feel?

10. On a scale from 0 (not very good at all) to 10 (I feel great!), how healthy are you?

11. Have you had any anti-aging procedures? If yes, which ones?

12. Do you exercise regularly? Have you found an enjoyable way to move your body so that you are more likely to exercise? What types of movement do you enjoy?

13. How do you want to feel about aging?

14. What specific actions do you need to take to feel good about aging? Can you list them?

Your Specific Desires and Goals for Aging

Here you will determine if you see yourself meeting your aging goal(s) and determine if you are the person you want to be?

1. What needs to change in your life for you to reach your goals and be the healthy person you want to be?

2. How much weight do you want to lose or what is your "perfect" weight—the weight in which you feel healthy and positive about yourself?

3. How do you want your body to shape up? Do you need to lift weights or do sit-ups to get there?

4. What clothes do you want to fit in and wear?

5. Are you comfortable with changes in your hair as you age?

6. How do you picture yourself in your 40s, 50s, 60s, and older?

7. If you experience a symptom related to aging issues like arthritis, what steps do you take to address it?

8. How much of "negative" aging do you think is overemphasized by society? Can you switch your thinking to positive aging?

9. How do you want people to react to you when they meet you for the first time?

10. How are you going to measure your success as you reach your healthy, victorious aging goals?

Aging is living at one point—your current health—and moving toward the destination that you desire. It's a journey that includes deciding, taking steps, and overcoming obstacles along the way. And just like planning a trip, you can plan how you would like to feel as your birthdays go by.

HISTORY

CHAPTER 2

In our society the elderly are regarded as biodegradable and superfluous, instead of what they really represent: a biological elite who, with weathered wisdom, have much to offer the world.

— Ashley Montagu

THE CURRENT OBSESSION with looking young didn't start yesterday. The word *vanity* dates to the thirteenth century and is associated with our obsession with beauty. Its Latin root, *vanitas*, means the quality of being empty or vain. It's also associated with a feeling of being valueless. Considering the meaning of the word, it's sad that vanity related to one's looks has become so prevalent today. Vanity branches off into other concepts: self-love, conceit, and *amour propre* (feelings of excessive pride and pridefulness). Its symbols include skulls, clocks, burning candles, and rotten fruit, all of which remind us of decay and the transient nature of life, earthly achievements, and pleasure. Only in still life artwork is the state of beauty static. For the living, the clock keeps ticking—no matter what method of anti-aging one chooses—and your body will age.

It's almost irrational that people frequently relate "premature aging" to the appearance of one wrinkle or line on their face at an early age. Changes in appearance as we age are natural and unavoidable. Hair grays. Skin becomes drier and less smooth.

You know about Narcissus, right? He was a beautiful boy but doomed because of his love for his own reflection. His first mirror was the reflective surface of still water. Narcissus's love for his own reflection is forever remembered in psychology as a pathology called *Narcissistic Personality Disorder*, characterized as an excessive need for admiration and affirmation. Narcissus's unrelenting love for his own reflection is still relevant because we have been looking in mirrors to find our *imperfections* since the invention of mirrors. Discs of polished obsidian served as the first mirrors. The Egyptian, Greek, and Roman people peered at themselves in mirrors made of polished metal. In the fifteenth century, colorless glass on a metallic background created a clearer reflection, and so the modern mirror was born.

The Cost of Beauty

Women have historically done crazy things to look younger and more beautiful. For over 4000 years, since the beginning of Chinese medicine, they've changed their appearance. Permanent makeup on mummies is evidence. Thousands of years ago, sculptures and artistic renditions of women were curvaceous. As time passed, the perfect female form turned from thicker to extremely thin. Skinny women like today's runway models became the beautiful ones. Mostly, the American standard of beauty has been unattainable.

Here are some things we've done to ourselves to fix imperfections or create a more beautiful image.

Nails

What was called "nail dye" originated in India, but "nail polish" originated in China when women soaked their nails in a combination of eggs whites, gelatin, beeswax, and dyes made from flower petals. Rose petals turn nails a reddish pink color, and the gelatin and beeswax added a shine. Sometimes they dusted the nails with gold or silver metallic dust. In Chinese history, upper-class women predominately wore color, and lower-class women were put to death for wearing the color of the royals. Cleopatra, who loved beauty and makeup, dipped her nails into blood red henna. The Aztecs and Incas decorated their fingernails with art. Now we have a rainbow of nail polish colors. There are also fake nails that require acids and chemicals to fix them in place. Unfortunately, the use of these substances can lead to fungal infections.

Lips

Early on, women crushed gemstones and blended them with oils and waxes to create lip color. Cleopatra used red ochre clay or mashed ants and carmine beetles in beeswax for her lip color. Others used human earwax as the waxy component. *Oh my!* Cleopatra's Egyptian counterparts applied a dangerous combination of highly toxic bromine mannite, iodine, and seaweed to their lips. As time went on, red dye, mulberries, mashed red beet roots, red iron oxide, red algae, fish scales, and wine residue became a popular mix for lip coloring. Sometimes these ingredients were mixed with sheep sweat, honey, human saliva, and even crocodile excrement. The Japanese used red safflower, water, and sugar crystals to create a lip gloss of sorts. Some say that Queen Elizabeth I invented the first lip pencil out of color and plaster of Paris. Despite its vacillation in popularity, Hollywood secured lipstick's place in the makeup world in the late 1800s. Now we're injecting lips, over plumping them even though lip injections can look unnatural and have negative side effects. We also tattoo color on lips. Oh, how far we have come.

Eyes

Egyptian men and women loved dramatic eye makeup. Their color concoctions were more or less harmful, containing lead, mercury, malachite, chrysocolla, or copper as key ingredients. People didn't think of it as dangerous; they applied eye makeup as if it was medicine. Some of the lead salt ingredients were indeed very dangerous, leading to brain and central nervous system damage. Kohl was used to darken lashes, eyelids, and eyebrows. For a less expensive blackening—and safer since kohl caused lead poisoning—they used the soot from burning candles. To create a wide-eyed seductive look during the Renaissance period, women used belladonna (*deadly nightshade*) eyedrops, which is as toxic as its name implies. Once again, Hollywood played a part in advancing the makeup industry because eyes had to "speak" in silent films. Modern government regulations now prevent the addition of toxic ingredients in cosmetics. We have advanced into eyelid surgery, eyebrow lifts, and Botox® injections that stop eyebrows from creating forehead lines.

Entire Complexion

Early cosmetic concoctions used lead dye to lighten the skin, but it often led to disfigurement and sometimes death. Just as awful, a mixture of carbonate, hydroxide, and lead oxide bleached the skin, resulting in muscle paralysis or death if used too often. Believe it or not, some women painted their skin with white lead paint to look lighter complected.

An ancient Egyptian medical text contained a recipe for a skin-rejuvenating acid peel that was much more skin friendly. Cleopatra used poultices made of milk to smooth her skin because lactic acid (an AHA still used in peels today) has skin smoothing properties. She even traveled with donkeys for a continuous supply of milk.

Another AHA in early chemical peels is tartaric acid, which is found in grapes or red wine. Citric acid, sulfur, and limestone were applied to skin to reduce age spots and minimize sun damage. Medical grade peels were developed in the late 1800s and included ingredients such as phenol, croton oil, salicylic acid, and nitric acid. These procedures were scary because the chemical formula was softened with boiling water, then brushed on the skin and bandaged for a few days. After removing the bandages/gauze, the result was a red, scabby face.

Today, there's a wide range of chemical potencies, and professionals study your skin type to choose the best blend to minimize burning, scarring, hyperpigmentation or hypopigmentation, and other unpleasant side effects.

Hair

Remember hearing "Only your hairdresser knows for sure?" Hairdressing and hair dyeing have been popular for centuries. Early hair dyes included chamomile, indigo, henna, sage, walnuts, leeks, black sulfur, honey, goat fat, and ashes. *The American Hairdresser* started its publication in 1877, and the turn of the century newspapers included ads for free hair and scalp food, specifically *Cranitonic Hair Food*. Some ads stated, "A woman is as old as she looks." They suggested you should buy Mrs. Potter's walnut juice hair stain. An electric hairbrush company claimed to remove dandruff, keep hair from falling out, and cure all scalp disorders. In 1928, A.B. Moler released *The Manual of Beauty Culture*. Beauty shops went into business and electric iron heaters were invented. Instructional books were published to teach how to create finger waves, water waves, moler waves, and more. Women were introduced to hairpins, hair nets, hair curlers, big hair, retro hair … Newly developed shampoos boasted they could produce styling miracles for the hair. Now we have all the colors in the rainbow for hair dyes, along with hair implants, extensions, relaxing formulas, and more.

These were all just a prelude to nose jobs in the 50s, breast augmentation in the 60s, and tummy tucks in the 70s. Today we undergo chin implants, hair replacement, pectoral resurrections, Gortex cheek implants, tattooed makeup, skin peels, lip injections and implants, spider threading, skin fillers, and a growing number of procedures that are used to hide the effects of aging.

Vanity reaches far beyond how we feel about our faces and hair. In some cultures, women bound their feet, as well as their breasts, to prevent being perceived as immoral. Before and during the Han Dynasty, a slender body was ideal, so began food deprivation. Then, in the Tang Dynasty, heavier women were in style, so the goal turned to gaining weight. Many cultures continue to send mixed messages about what is attractive, especially regarding body weight. Which is it: thin or heavy? It's important for everyone to have an inner sense of personal beauty and value rather than complying with fads.

Victorious Aging from the Inside Out

Over 2000 years ago, women in Chinese medicine used acupuncture for anti-aging. They also believed that treating the internal organs and meridians (acupuncture channels) affected their appearance. In other words, treating the inside reflects on the outside. According to Chinese medicine, each organ system controls some aspect of beauty. The lungs control the skin and body hair; they also affect the moisture of the skin. The spleen's balanced energy can naturally affect the skin and lips. If your heart energy is disturbed, you may lose sleep and end up having dark circles under your eyes. It makes sense to stay healthy on the inside to look healthy on the outside.

As far back as 1121–770 B.C. medical books included information about food and herbal recommendations for the skin. Soon after that, instructions about herbal masks were added to the texts. *Materia Medica*, written during the Ming dynasty, addressed specific parts of the face and ways to address the complexion and wrinkles.

There are lifestyles, traditions, and medical systems, like the ones I practice with TCM, that support attaining youthfulness and beauty. They engage in *victorious aging* from the inside out by committing to living a healthy lifestyle and minimizing the effects of the ticking clock. A basic tenet of TCM is that your outside reflects the status of your health on the inside. In Chinese medicine, health is all about balance and harmony. It is the balance of yin and yang, and the free flow of energy through your body that helps keep your face and skin vibrant and your weight at a healthy level. Ask yourself, is your digestion in balance? Do you have issues with bloating, acid reflux, feeling too full when you eat just a little, or irregular bowel movements? These are symptoms that your digestion is not working up to par. Believe it or not, good digestion helps your skin appear healthy and vibrant. It's a good example of literally seeing beauty from the inside out.

In modern times, people have forgotten that beauty and a youthful appearance come from within. They've forgotten that looking young is a part of having a healthy inside. Most cosmetic procedures only address the outside and some may be bad for your health. The most effective way to achieve and maintain a youthful appearance is to work from the inside out or work on both the inside and the outside in ways that are natural and safe. How do you work on the inside? Schedule an appointment for acupuncture or a massage. Evaluate your diet and nutritional intake. See your doctor.

Modern advancements in anti-aging technologies are doing their best to go natural, including the study of drugs that can reprogram our T cells to turn them into aging-cell-killing T cells. The biological mechanisms of aging—the development of conditions like diabetes and dementia—drive the research on drugs that may mitigate aging mechanisms. So, the next step might be an anti-aging pill.

Another area of anti-aging research is to reinforce longevity and prevent disease onset, preserving good health. Geroscience studies aging as a modifiable disease. Life expectancies are getting older, 84.3 years for men and 86.6 years for women. Throughout our life span we can exercise, learn new things, be happy, live independently, and, with care, look vibrant.

I have many patients who are using Mei Zen Cosmetic Acupuncture as their anti-aging cosmetic procedure for their face and neck. Even younger women in their 30s are exhibiting results from cosmetic acupuncture. Their friends ask what they're doing to their skin because of the visible improvements in their skin's texture and tone. Older women, like Bonnie, a patient in her 60s, has people asking her how she continues to look so youthful. It's because she receives regular monthly cosmetic acupuncture treatments, takes care of her skin with natural products, and always wears sunscreen.

Or consider Donna, who receives regular acupuncture to stay well. She uses Chinese medicine as her "true anti-aging medicine" because when your health is strong, you age more gracefully. That is, when your general health is robust, you look more vibrant. With robust general health, you are less likely to suffer through colds or flu that use up qi, which negatively impacts aging. It's all about maintenance: maintaining good health inside and maintaining your skin's health from inside and outside.

For some people, there may come a time when a cosmetic procedure becomes more or less necessary. Let's say that someone has a bit of ptosis (the eyelid droops over the eye). Surgery would tighten the muscle to raise the eyelid. Botox® is another non-surgical option—going from invasive surgery to a much less invasive injection. There are also eyedrops for mild cases of ptosis. For saggy neck skin, options range from a surgical neck lift to less invasive laser treatments or a healthier choice like cosmetic acupuncture. We have choices.

Your Beauty and Anti-Aging History Checklist

Here are some thoughtful questions that can help you reflect on your personal history with beauty aids and anti-aging techniques. These questions encourage introspection and discussion, like those in Chapter 1.

Your Experience

1. What was your first experience with beauty aids or anti-aging products? How did it make you feel?

2. Can you recall any beauty practices or products that were popular in your family or culture when you were growing up? Did you use any of them?

3. Have you ever felt pressured by society, media, or peers to use certain beauty aids or undergo anti-aging procedures? How did you respond to that pressure?

4. What are some beauty aids or anti-aging techniques you've tried in the past? Were they effective or disappointing?

5. How has your perception of beauty and aging changed over the years?

6. Do you have any beauty rituals that you follow regularly? How do they make you feel?

7. Have you ever experienced negative side effects from any beauty aids or anti-aging treatments? How did you handle the situation?

8. Are there any traditional or cultural beauty practices you find particularly interesting or effective?

9. How do you balance the use of beauty aids with maintaining a healthy lifestyle?

10. What do you think about the portrayal of beauty and aging in modern media? How does it influence your choices regarding beauty aids and anti-aging?

11. Have you ever consulted with a professional (i.e., dermatologist or cosmetic acupuncturist) about your beauty or anti-aging concerns? What was the experience like?

12. Do you believe that certain beauty aids or anti-aging treatments can make you feel younger or more confident? Why or why not?

13. How important is it for you to use natural or organic beauty products? Do you notice a difference when you use them?

14. What are your goals when using beauty aids or anti-aging treatments? Are they more about appearance, confidence, health, or something else?

15. How do you feel about the balance between inner health and outer beauty? Do you think one is more important than the other?

16. How has your use of beauty aids and anti-aging products evolved?

17. What lessons have you learned from your experiences with various beauty and anti-aging techniques?

18. Do you have any beauty or anti-aging goals for the future? What steps are you taking to achieve them?

19. How do you define beauty for yourself? How has this definition changed since you've aged?

20. If you could give one piece of advice to your younger self about beauty and aging, what would it be?

Your Action Steps

1. Make a list of beauty aids or anti-aging products you currently use. Evaluate their effectiveness and how they make you feel.

2. Consider trying a new beauty or anti-aging technique that aligns with your values and health goals.

3. Reflect on a beauty practice from your cultural heritage that you haven't tried yet. How might incorporating it into your routine benefit you?

4. Set a goal to improve an aspect of your inner health (e.g., nutrition, exercise, stress management) and observe how it affects your outer beauty.

SKIN

CHAPTER 3

Wrinkles here and there seem unimportant
compared to the Gestalt of the whole person I
have become in this past year.

– May Sarton

Let's talk about your skin and be frank about one of our main aging concerns: wrinkles.

Skin begins aging when you're much younger than you think. When we're young, and our skin is smooth and our tan is flawless, we think little about taking extra steps to help preserve that smooth, even-toned, wrinkle-free look. We imagine it will last forever. We really do take our skin for granted. Or maybe we figure we'll deal with wrinkles and sagging when the time comes, but it seems so far into the future. Well, from my professional experience in treating wrinkles, it is easier to prevent wrinkles than erase them, so start preventing wrinkles early. Wrinkle prevention includes putting on sunscreen every day, even when you're young. Moms should put sunscreen on children every day they go out to play.

When I was a master sunbathing teenager, I didn't consider sunscreen. And that's my excuse for the sun damage that occurred to my skin as a younger person. But now I know better and implore every young person to take care of their skin early, early, early. This is because every time you are under the sun without sunscreen, your skin is further damaged. The sun is the #1 cause of wrinkles. Yes, the #1 cause. Repeated sunburn and prolonged exposure to the radiation from sunlight causes irreparable damage to the DNA of skin cells. Melanoma is one of the most rapidly increasing forms of cancer, and unprotected exposure to the ultraviolet rays of the sun is the most preventable risk factor.

Collagen and Elastin

Collagen and elastin are the goddesses of smooth skin. How do they work and what happens to them as we age?

Collagen is one of the main proteins in skin that gives it strength and elasticity. As collagen declines with age, skin sags and wrinkles. The production of collagen and elastin declines in our 30s, and the firm and supple skin that we enjoy so much in our twenties shows signs of aging.

Unfortunately, you can't just use a collagen cream to improve your collagen production. For wrinkles to disappear or improve, topical collagen must penetrate the layers of skin that are called the dermis. The collagen molecules in many creams are too large to penetrate through the epidermis—the outer layers of skin—to make it into the dermis below. The epidermis' outer layer alone (the stratum corneum) has 15 to 40 layers of flattened skin cells that move up from deeper layers and replace themselves about once a month. It's our natural exfoliation process. This barrier helps keep moisture from escaping and would, conversely, prevent larger molecules like collagen from getting in. One layer beneath is keratinocytes, followed by Langerhans cells and melanocytes. These cells protect the dermis below and any cream would have to make it through all the above layers to get to the dermis. The fact is that only stimulation of the skin cells in the dermis itself will activate fibroblasts to improve collagen production.

What is the perfect dermis stimulating tool? The acupuncture needle! It's true. From the Chinese medicine perspective, facial needling causes oxygen and blood to rise to the face to lift the skin and improve the quality of the skin and fascia. From a Western medicine perspective, the potential to improve collagen formation occurs when the acupuncture needles inflict what are called *micro-traumas* in the skin. When the skin perceives a trauma or wound, fibroblasts of collagen and elastin rush to the site to heal it. The body's wound healing process involves collagen and elastin. Think about how a cut heals to make your skin whole again. It's the same process. A scar is an overgrowth of collagen and elastin. The dermis produces collagen, so to boost its production, you need a procedure or product that reaches beyond the epidermis and targets the dermis directly. That's why your collagen and elastin cells are more abundant after the needling. Preventing or reducing collagen breakdown and increasing its supply are the only ways to minimize wrinkling and sagging.

Unfortunately, as we age, our skin loses its capability to replace damaged collagen, which is why we need procedures like acupuncture to boost collagen repair. And any cosmetic procedure that claims to have permanent results must impact collagen. For said results to last, the process requires multiple treatments over weeks for the matrix of collagen and elastin to grow. As far as I know, there are no immediate or one-treatment cosmetic procedures that give long-lasting results. Well, a surgical facelift is a one-treatment procedure that lasts for several years, but it's one of the more drastic procedures available. Bottom line, no cosmetic procedure is permanent, even a surgical facelift. The clock keeps ticking; we keep aging; changes happen.

Skin in Your 30s

If you are in your 30s, your skin has already worsened, even if you are not yet seeing any visible signs of aging. When I teach Cosmetic Acupuncture, I use the nickname "the decade of decline" for our skin in our 30s. This is prime time to focus on prevention, and why it is so important to start natural wrinkle prevention treatments like Cosmetic Acupuncture. It's a lot easier to prevent a wrinkle than it is to make it go away. I always try to influence thirty-somethings to receive Cosmetic Acupuncture treatments to prevent or at least decelerate wrinkling as long as possible. If you are in your early 30s and don't see any lines or wrinkles—I'm not kidding—now is the time to begin prevention treatments. Here are some reasons to take better care of your skin:

- One issue with our 30-year-old skin is the significant reduction of oil production. This creates the need to moisturize your skin regularly.

- Skin's natural exfoliation process slows in our 30s. Instead of cells sloughing off dead skin every 28 days, it takes about 40 days. The longer the dead cells remain in the epidermis, the duller our skin looks. I've seen women in their 70s and 80s whose skin appears gray, and it's because they never exfoliate. Exfoliate means removing those layers of dead skin cells with an exfoliating product or procedure.

- Production of our naturally produced plumping sugar, hyaluronic acid, decreases in our 30s and continues to decrease as we grow older. This is because the synthesis of hyaluronic acid is a complex process, and the metabolic power of our cells gradually degrades with age. Lower amounts of hyaluronic acid result in skin losing hydration, volume, and plumpness.

- The average age for first pregnancies was once 27, but birthrates have risen for women in their 30s. It's no surprise that pregnancy and childbearing can change skin. Often, pregnant women have a "pregnancy glow" because of increased blood flow and oil production. But increased oil production can lead to acne. Another issue that occurs during pregnancy is dark spots or darkened areas that look like a mask. It fades a few months after giving birth, but use sunscreen during pregnancy to help prevent any darkening. Increased blood volume and hormonal changes during pregnancy can cause tiny red veins on your face and/or neck. Again, they usually clear up after pregnancy. Last but not least, hormones released during pregnancy cause hair growth on unwanted places such as the face or neck.

Many of us are working hard at our careers in our 30s. You may not think that sitting behind a desk all day can hurt your skin, but it really does. When you sit all day, your blood pumps more slowly, depleting vital nutrients and oxygen from your body. The reduction in nutrients contributes to the premature aging of the skin. Staying sedentary can also raise your risk of developing acne and worsen existing skin conditions. It also plays a role in increasing sebum production and/or inflammation so your skin is oilier. We all know that too much oil clogs pores and triggers blemishes and acne. And too much inactivity indoors increases the risk of anxiety and depression.

Recommended Actions

While we experience many changes to our skin in our 30s, there are things you can do to mitigate aging.

- Moisturize in the morning and evening.

- Place your moisturizer on moist skin.

- Apply a moisturizing mask at least once a week.

- Read skin care labels and use products that contain nutrients such as vitamin C and vitamin E.

- Exfoliate your skin regularly. Try procedures such as microdermabrasion from a qualified professional or natural products like foaming scrubs.

Homemade Skin Care

There are lots of natural ways to help your skin look its best at any age:

- Simple at-home moisturizers include egg yolks, blueberries, papaya, and avocado. Yes, whole food masks are great! Just mash up the whole food, add a little honey, and apply the mix for a wonderful moisturizing mask.

- Apple cider vinegar exfoliates the skin, increasing the skin's cell cycle. It also balances skin's pH levels.

- Raw honey is nourishing and anti-bacterial, so it's good for people who experience acne breakouts. And it's moisturizing, not drying.

Skin in Your 40s

Your dermis thins in your 40s. The outer few layers of skin are called your epidermis, and it's about four pieces of paper thick and composed of mainly dead skin cells. The deeper layers of the epidermis contain live cells, but those cells do not have the regenerative properties that the cells in your dermis possess. Underneath the epidermis is the dermis, and it can be as thick as forty sheets of paper, although the thickness varies widely. Your dermis is where the money is. It's the central nervous system or brain of the skin. It's where stimulation must occur for the most effective, long-lasting cosmetic results. So, your 40s is the time to treat the dermis before it gets too thin.

The need to moisturize and exfoliate speeds up during your 40s because of the continued skin degradation processes. *Sigh.* Hormonal changes prevent our skin from retaining adequate moisture, causing drier skin and the need to moisturize. These hormonal changes also produce more age spots, cause uneven tanning, and lead to breakouts. Hot flashes can also redden skin. Our skin feels "the change" as well as the rest of our body.

Despite this, perimenopause and menopause are not bad times or horrible events. When we were 7-year-olds, we didn't have periods; when we were 11 or 12 or 13, we did. Menstruation didn't make our lives an awful thing. It was our life; we dealt with it. Having a period was a new part of life. It's the same with perimenopause and menopause. Frankly, I almost wish they didn't have labels because the words are so stigmatized. Some Chinese medicine books call menopause "Second Spring" and suggest it is a time of personal growth and a chance to nurture yourself. Speaking of labels, if we called the "chore" of self-care nurturing or pampering, maybe we would be happier about taking care of ourselves.

One of my patients asked me to join a Facebook community for women in perimenopause and menopause because she thought I could provide some value on how to transition through it. You know what happened? I had to take a break from the group a week after joining because every post complained about the tortures of perimenopause. I doubted how great I felt, how pleased I was with my weight, how well I could run … How could I be the only one? Our bodies change, but it's not luck that I'm healthy. True, I use Chinese medicine—the true anti-aging medicine. Did I have any issues, like insomnia for example? Yes, but I follow my own advice and take steps similar to these to deal with it.

Recommended Actions

If you're in your 40s and changes are happening, *relax*. Perimenopause is a stage in a woman's life. You are liable to spend more than half of your life in perimenopause and menopause—enjoy it!

- There are lots of practices (pampering) you should follow: moisturize, exercise, stay hydrated, get enough sleep, meditate, chant, breathe … Hmm, these are ideas for every stage of life!

- A complaint I get in the clinic with perimenopausal women is that they are sleeping less (insomnia) or suffering from poor quality sleep. Sleep is important for our immune system, mood, and skin because during sleep, our cells recover from the damage that they experienced during the day. When suffering from chronic sleep deficiency, skin's protective barrier decreases its ability to maintain moisture, which can lead to drier skin. Keep sleep aids nearby, including things like chamomile tea, calming mantras, self-hypnosis/hypnosis for sleep recordings, and this simple breathing exercise (breathe in to the count of 5, out to the count of 7, pause/hold for 3, then repeat several times).

Skin in Your 50s

In your 50s, you will notice deeper lines and wrinkles. By now, your dermis has become even thinner, and you may look a little saggy. It's time to prevent the neck wattle. Once we reach perimenopause or menopause, things change in our body again. Estrogen Replacement Therapy (ERT) helps stave off skin changes, but ERT isn't for everyone. Without hormone therapy, your skin will further dry. Remember, decreased oil and hyaluronic acid production started in your 30s. The slower skin cell turnover that started twenty years prior also exacerbates dryness. And skin is even thinner because of lower estrogen.

An interesting change you may notice in your 50s is that your skin is more sensitive. This is partly because of reduced lipids, our natural moisture, but also because the pH level of skin increases, making us prone to rashes, dermatitis, and general sensitivity. I must stress again that proper moisturizing can help with this too.

Studies in Occupational Medicine have reported that people become more sedentary as they age. Approximately one in four adults over 50 are inactive and the prevalence of inactivity is higher among women than men. This is interesting to me because I became more active as I aged. In fact, I block out time in my schedule to run or walk or bike. Maybe it's because, as a healthcare provider and one who has studied cardiovascular disease in my early career, I know the importance of exercise. Find an activity that you enjoy because it's important for you to keep movement in your healthcare routine.

Funny story, I used to play soccer and loved everything about it: running fast, the competition, and the camaraderie with my friends. I ran during the week between games because I believed my muscles needed to stay strong so I could run fast on the soccer pitch. When people said, "You must love running," I replied, "No, I hate it. I only run to get faster on the soccer field." Well, during the pandemic, playing soccer changed as did many other activities. I continued to run instead of competing in soccer. The thing that I always said I hated to do turned out to be what I love to do! I took running lessons, found proper shoes, and bought proper attire. I now run at least 3 days a week. So, we *can* change!

Our 50s may require more action and more "dramatic" skin care. At the very least, the products you use must contain essential oils along with natural active cosmeceuticals to help the moisturizing ingredients work. Products should include important active ingredients like AHAs, plant stem cells, peptides, and enzymes along with essential oils that all come together to support, renew, and regenerate your skin.

It's never too late to help your skin! I have treated women who are in their eighties with Cosmetic Acupuncture and know from experience that it's never too late to have healthier, younger-looking skin, as well as to feel your best. Naturally, the older you are and the longer you have worn your wrinkles, lines, or sagging, the more subtle your results may be. On the other hand, those may be the people who get the most dramatic results!

Recommended Actions

Your skin's going to continue aging, but you can fend off the visible signs of aging by using my recommended actions. And there are many procedures or treatments to choose from, but I recommend reading about their potential side effects. Some side effects are very mild, others are serious. Your dermatologist may offer procedures like chemical peels, microneedling (some acupuncturists also offer this), fat injections, dermal fillers, Botox® injections, dermaplaning, laser resurfacing, acne blue light therapy, Thermage, microdermabrasion, and more. These procedures do anything from making your skin cleaner and more vibrant to filling up lines and wrinkles. Still, these are the best skin care procedures:

- Cleanse both in the morning and evening.

- Tone in the morning and evening.

- Treat/moisturize with a cream or serum morning and evening. Use specialty products around your eyes.

- Exfoliate once or twice a week.

- Mask once or twice a week.

- Protect every day with sunscreen.

- Be nice to your skin!

Finally, you can add these routines to your regimen:

- Shorten hot showers because they lead to drier skin.

- Pat your skin dry after showering or bathing rather than rubbing it dry. Also leave a little water on your skin.

- Commit to wearing sunscreen every day no matter your age!

- Exfoliate to promote circulation in your skin and brighten your complexion.

- Reduce sugar intake because it causes inflammation and damages collagen.

- Pay attention to your digestion. In Chinese medicine, when patients improve digestion, their skin looks better. Your gut microbiome affects your skin and your general health, heart health, and brain health. It's important to have good digestion.

- Use products with vitamin C and/or retinol.

Practices and Habits That Prematurely Age Your Skin

This is a good time to mention ways of prematurely aging your skin. I've already mentioned many times that excessive sun exposure, especially without applying the proper sunscreen, accelerates the appearance of wrinkles, dark spots, and loose skin. Smoking reduces collagen and leads to more sagging. If you eat a diet high in sugar and other processed foods, you'll experience a breakdown of collagen. Even how much water you drink affects your skin: dehydrated skin makes fine lines more prominent. Let's look at these aging factors in more detail.

Smoking

Besides being bad for your general health, smoking is bad for your skin. The chemicals in the cigarettes themselves and their smoke wreak havoc on your skin both internally and externally.

Nicotine reduces vascularization in the dermis, depriving your skin of oxygen. Smoking also increases enzymes that lead to the degradation of collagen. Second-hand smoke is just as bad. And the inhalation of smoke forms deeper lines around the lips.

Quit smoking to improve your skin and minimize lines around your lips. Seek help from professionals or programs if needed. Acupuncture treatments are helpful for smoking cessation.

Air Pollution

Skin is an organ in direct contact with various air pollutants. There is a direct association between air pollution and damaging effects on the skin. Studies on the effect of ozone on cutaneous tissue show that ozone is an oxidative agent capable of affecting the integrity of the skin. A recent epidemiological study discovered a direct link between airborne particulates from pollution and the occurrence of age spots and wrinkles.

I won't suggest you move to the country where the air is cleaner. You live where you live. What can you do if you live in a polluted city? Take care of your skin the best you can: cleanse, tone, moisturize. Use a good cleanser and do an occasional mask to keep your skin clean and healthy. Protect your skin by using antioxidant-rich skin care products that help neutralize the damage caused by pollutants. And consider using a good air purifier at home.

The Sun

Do you have a history of sunbathing? If so, as I mentioned earlier, your skin is sun damaged. The process is called photo-aging. Sun is the #1 external factor that creates lines and wrinkles. People look older than they are because of sun damage to skin cells. Sun exposure decreases elasticity and causes skin to sag. Skin becomes drier and rougher, and growths like keratoses (liver or age spots) appear. Sun damage causes the blood capillaries in the dermis to decrease while making others dilated, dark red, and noticeable. For the most part, sun damage is irreversible because UV rays damage the skin's DNA. There is no such thing as an *anti-aging suntan.*

Twenty minutes a day in the sun while protecting your delicate facial, neck, and décolleté skin is an adequate daily dose of vitamin D. You *must, must, must* wear sunscreen—one that protects from both UVB and UVA rays. It's not an option; it's required. Living in Colorado, I enjoy the high-altitude sun, but my face, neck, and décolleté are always protected by sunblock and a hat, especially if I plan to spend extended time in the great outdoors.

Alcohol Use

Drinking alcohol dehydrates your skin, leading to a loss of elasticity and an increased risk of sagging and redness. Dry skin can look dull and gray, and dry skin wrinkles quicker than moist skin. The diuretic effect of alcohol also causes your skin to lose vitamins and nutrients like vitamin A.

Too much sugar also leads to sagging skin. Your body can only properly process so much sugar. Alcoholic drinks have high sugar content. Think about the amount of sugar in a margarita. High sugar content in alcoholic drinks can also lead to glycation, a process that damages collagen. In Chinese medicine, healthy spleen channel energy keeps things lifted. Too many sweets or too much sugar depletes spleen channel energy, which leads to sagging.

Limit alcohol intake to maintain skin hydration and overall health, especially if your skin is saggy or reddish. Opt for lower sugar drinks and always drink plenty of water to stay hydrated.

Coffee Consumption

Do you drink a pot of coffee a day? Like alcohol, caffeine is a diuretic and therefore contributes to making your skin too dry and lacking in nutrients. It can also interfere with sleep, which is crucial for skin regeneration. In TCM, we know that a woman's yin (the moisturizing part of the yin/yang pair) declines with age. This causes hot flashes during perimenopause and sometimes even after menopause. Drinking too much caffeine exacerbates that deficiency. I drink coffee, I just don't overdo it or drink it all day long. Sometimes more isn't better.

Cut down on coffee if you notice that your skin is dry or red or scaly. You can substitute herbal teas or other caffeine-free beverages to help maintain hydration.

Harsh Soaps

Harsh soaps contain chemicals and a much higher pH than skin. Anything above pH 11 is too high for use on the skin. Using an abrasive soap can lead to dehydrated, dry, irritated skin. Most traditional bar soaps strip the skin of moisture, leading to dryness and irritation. Harsh soap also contains harmful fragrance and chemicals that bind the soap. Soaps that irritate skin clog pores and cause acne breakouts.

Don't put bar soap directly on your face, neck, or décolleté. If your skin feels tight after washing, it may mean that the soap you are using is too drying. Switch to a gentle, moisturizing skin care regimen that contains hydrating ingredients like glycerin or hyaluronic acid. Moisturizing cleansers support your skin's natural barrier.

Poor Digestion

Poor gut health means your skin won't receive the nutrition it needs. Proper digestion affects your face in two ways: 1) it allows you to access ingested nutrients, and 2) it reflects in your skin through moisture and luster. Poor digestion, unhealthy gut, or "leaky gut" creates autoimmune responses that lead to irritated skin, rashes, and breakouts. This is because the imbalance in your gut bacteria has a negative influence on your skin. Poor digestion can even lead to an overall breakdown of collagen. For example, inflammatory bowel disease (IBD), psoriasis, and eczema are related.

Focus on eating real, whole foods. Eat probiotics like kimchi and sauerkraut. Also eat prebiotic foods like onions, oatmeal, and asparagus. Remove inflammatory foods from your diet. Eat more fiber because it helps feed the gut bacteria. And ask your acupuncturist how acupuncture can improve your digestive system.

Stress

We often hear that stress is bad for you. Well, the effects of stress on the body and health are negative for sure. But stress is just life. Hans Selye said, "Stress is the spice of life; the absence of stress is death." This means that stress will always be there in some form or another and our body will react. It reacts to any changes, threats, or pressures that come from outside sources. Then it tries to regain its normal state and continue to protect itself from potential harm. Dealing with stress is a process.

Stress can be cumulative, especially when it's repeated or chronic. The accumulation of stress may eventually result in damage to your general health and susceptibility to mental health issues like depression. Common dermatological issues like acne, rosacea, psoriasis, and hives are worse when you are under excessive stress. Anxiety and stress can cause conditions like eczema to flare up. You know the saying, "hot and bothered"? Well, if stress makes you "hot and bothered" it can also make your skin red and itchy or create hives, aka "stress rash."

On the other side, having a skin condition may lead to anxiety, depression, lower self-confidence, and reduced quality of life. It can become a vicious cycle. Plus, from a purely physical standpoint, stress triggers the release of hormones such as adrenaline and cortisol that lead to inflammation and acne. There's a branch of psychology called psychodermatology, but one of my patients preferred to call her therapist a "skin-emotion specialist." Psychodermatologists study the connection between stress and skin conditions, exploring how emotional well-being affects the skin. Their research has led to effective interventions such as biofeedback, cognitive-behavioral therapy, guided imagery, and hypnosis. These treatments offer hope for those struggling with stress-induced skin issues or the emotional toll caused by chronic skin conditions.

Our bodies have been under stress since the beginning of human existence. For ancient man, the threats were more physical such as animal attacks, hunger, and fire. We were just trying to stay alive. Today, the mind manufactures much of our stress, meaning that we fear our partner is angry with us, we're going to miss a deadline, or we can't pay a bill. But our bodies lack the ability to discern a deadline from a tiger at the door, and so our body responds with the same stress response or distress that it has forever. If we don't cope well, the stress response continues and our bodies cannot regulate back to normal, which can lead to negative health or skin consequences.

Stress has a negative impact on skin and can cause the following damage:

- Sebaceous glands excrete more oil, leading to breakouts.

- Hormones release, encouraging the lining of hair follicles to thicken, causing blackheads and whiteheads. The resulting inflammation may also be related to rosacea.

- Blood vessels constrict or dilate abnormally, causing too little or too much blood flow to the skin. Your face will either appear flushed or pale.

- Inflammatory neuropeptides release into the skin, making it more sensitive.

Address the source of stress and take good care of your body. Is the cause of your stress something under your control (like your credit card debt) or out of your control (like terrorism)? If the cause is something that is out of your control, let it go or do something about it. If the cause is in your control, then address it.

QiGong

Find ways to relax, regenerate, and get back on track. *QiGong* is a non-religious, natural, mental, and physical way to relax and regenerate. And it doesn't require any special equipment or location. Qi means "energy" and gong means "practice." It's a simple, gentle, and safe form of energetic exercise that is effective for relaxation, meditation, and physical fitness.

Follow these guidelines when doing a QiGong maneuver:

1. Use natural breathing. Inhale through your nose like you usually do. The nose is the gateway to the lungs, where the Heavenly Qi of air enters, so the nose plays a part in absorbing

the Qi. There is no need to think about your breathing or follow a rhythm, just breathe naturally.

2. Take a standing or sitting position/posture when doing these exercises. Be comfortable.

3. Place the tip of your tongue against the back of your front upper teeth, into the natural placement of your tongue when your mouth is closed. Again, don't stress about exact placement.

4. Close your eyes so you can concentrate.

5. Imagine there is a figure 8 infinity symbol, the top being level with your chest and the bottom level with your lower belly, below your navel.

6. Put your hands on your lower belly in a comfortable position.

7. Breathe normally and think about that figure 8 infinity symbol, connecting your upper and lower body and the gentle flow of energy in your body.

This connection delivers good energy so that your digestion works well, spirit is calm, demeanor is relaxed, stress level is minimized, and your energy is strong and moves to all our extremities to help relieve pain, edema, etc.

A bonus is that your body remembers how pleasant balance feels, making it better able to react and recover from stressors in shorter periods of time.

Exercises for Your Face

1. Place both your hands close to your face but not touching it.

2. "Rub" above your face from top to bottom, then bottom to top using little circles. Do this 20-30 times until you feel warmth or heat in your hands and/or on your face.

3. Gently massage your temples with your fingertips in a circular motion. Again, do it for 20-30 circles.

4. Place your palms over your ears with your thumbs in the indentations at the base/back of your skull. Spread the rest of your fingers along the back and sides of your head. With your little fingers facing up, tap the back of your head 20-30 times and imagine how the Qi is pulling up from the sides of your face to the top of your head.

5. Massage the inner part of your eyebrows at the top of your nose in a circular movement.

6. Massage the slight indentation right below your lower eyelid with your index fingers and form small circles.

7. Use little circular movements to massage next to your nostrils.

Regular use of these short techniques will allow your body to stay balanced and recover faster from stress or physical illness.

Understanding how to care for your skin through the various stages of life is crucial for maintaining its health and vitality. By being mindful of the factors that contribute to premature aging and taking proactive steps to support your skin's natural functions, you will enjoy a more youthful and radiant appearance at any age. Remember, the key to beautiful skin lies in a combination of internal health and external care. Embrace a holistic approach, and your skin will thank you.

Chinese Medicine and Skin

Chinese medicine believes that skin conditions are linked to dysfunction of the organ systems, of yin and yang, of heat and cold, or the result of other imbalances, including emotional stress. Stress or imbalances in any of the organ systems don't stay confined to one place and, since the skin is our largest organ, it is easily affected by disharmony. For example, less Yin (the cool, more fluid part of the yin yang pair) leads to symptoms of dryness or heat. This may be one reason skin gets drier during perimenopause. According to the theory of Chinese medicine, yin depletion is common during perimenopause and menopause. On the other hand, yang imbalances may lead to inflammatory skin issues, including rosacea and acne. While skin issues originate from imbalances inside the body, there are also ways to treat skin issues from the outside using Chinese medicine. Herbal masks, facial Gua Sha, and Cosmetic Acupuncture are all helpful in treating a variety of skin conditions.

Reader Reflection Questions

1. At what age did you first become concerned about wrinkles or signs of aging? What prompted your concern?

2. How consistent are you with using sunscreen?

3. Has your skin care routine changed over the years?

4. What brands of skin care products do you use regularly? Do you pay attention to their ingredients and how they affect your skin?

5. Have you tried any procedures or treatments aimed at reducing wrinkles or improving skin texture? What were your experiences and results?

6. How do you feel about natural versus cosmetic approaches to skin care? Which do you prefer and why?

7. Do you have a skin care routine that includes moisturizing and exfoliating?

8. How does your diet and lifestyle affect your skin? Have you noticed any particular foods or habits that make a significant difference?

9. Have you experienced any skin issues related to stress? What strategies have you found effective for managing stress and its impact on your skin?

10. How do you perceive your skin's health and appearance compared to others your age? What influences your perception?

Action Steps

1. Assess your current skin care routine and identify areas for improvement.

2. Make a plan to incorporate more holistic practices into your skin care regimen, such as regular acupuncture, healthy diet changes, or stress management techniques.

3. Set a goal to reduce or eliminate habits that contribute to premature aging, like smoking or excessive alcohol consumption.

4. Commit to daily sunscreen use and find a product that suits your skin type and lifestyle.

5. Explore natural ingredients and DIY skin care recipes that complement your existing routine and provide additional benefits.

NUTRITION AND SKIN HEALTH

CHAPTER 4

Age is simply the number of years the world has been enjoying you.

– Author Unknown

W E'VE ALL HEARD advice on preventing premature skin aging and maintaining a youthful appearance. One key factor is nutrition—eating a healthy, well-balanced diet. Many chronic diseases linked to aging are preventable with proper nutrition and lifestyle choices. In fact, a significant number of cancers are associated with diet and smoking. Try to reduce emotional eating, as it often leads to poor food choices and overeating. Instead, manage stress through meditation, walking, or chanting. Also, avoid processed foods, which provide little nutrition and are often high in sugar and sodium.

Nutritional therapy in TCM maintains a healthy body and relieves symptoms or illness when they happen. It can also slow down the aging process.

It's believed that one can balance yin and yang using food as medicine. There are several classic texts about the effects of nutrition on health. *Plain Questions: On Soup and Mash* is one such text, focusing on boiling grains into soups and mashes. This boiling technique makes grains easier to digest, strengthens the digestive system, and helps nourish both yin and yang. Soups and mashes are especially beneficial for supporting the spleen and stomach, which are key to maintaining overall health and vitality in Chinese medicine.

Just as balance is crucial in the yin-yang relationship, it is equally important to maintain a well-rounded diet of grains, fruits, vegetables, and what the Chinese refer to as "livestock." Digestion functions best with warm foods, while cold or iced foods force the digestive system to work harder, potentially hindering nutrient absorption. If someone is experiencing a heat-related condition, such as inflammation or acne, they should avoid hot, energetically warming foods for optimal results.

TCM also incorporates "flavor prescriptions" to support overall balance. For example, excessive salt intake can disrupt kidney qi, weaken bones, and depress heart qi. Similarly, individuals prone to bloating are advised to limit overly bitter foods.

As you can see, food therapy balances yin and yang using the energetics, flavors, and temperatures of the foods that are prescribed for the individual's condition. "Going on a diet" in Chinese medicine means nourishing the body using the principle of balance.

Chinese medicine food therapy has identified foods that help stave off skin aging, improve the elasticity of facial tissue, and help reduce the production of wrinkles. Here's what you can do in the world of food to maintain a vibrant, healthy life and, as a result, maintain healthy skin and a youthful appearance.

Using Food as Medicine

According to TCM theory, foods have specific energies, affect certain organs or acupuncture channel systems, and relieve a variety of symptoms or conditions. Food is medicine that is consumed several times a day.

There are even foods we recommend for particular skin or health issues. For example, some foods encourage growth of healthy skin and improve collagen and elastin. Spinach, apples, and sesame seeds encourage the growth of skin tissue. Apricots, Asian pears, and cherries also generate body fluids, making them excellent skin moisturizing foods. Kale and lemons also aid in tissue regeneration. Here are some other foods you should add to your diet.

Cruciferous Vegetables

How are cruciferous vegetables beneficial to you? They contain phytonutrients that detox the liver of the harmful chemicals we encounter daily. And these vegetables have been studied for their cancer-preventing properties. They have anti-inflammatory effects, induce cell death (apoptosis), and inhibit tumor blood vessel formation and the tumor cell migration that is needed for metastasis. The American Institute of Cancer Research also says that a molecule in these vegetables inactivates a gene that plays a role in some cancers.

Cruciferous vegetables include arugula, broccoli, brussels sprouts, cabbage, cauliflower, kale, radishes, and turnips.

Berries

Berries contain phytochemicals and vitamin C. They also contain ellagic acid that fights skin damage caused by the sun and the breakdown of collagen and elastic.

Blueberries are an excellent source of vitamin C, vitamin K, and manganese. They improve digestion because they are prebiotics, fighting gut inflammation and dysbiosis. Wild blueberries win as the most antioxidant-rich berry with vitamins A, C, K, and flavonoids like quercetin and polyphenols that help reduce cholesterol and the overall risk for heart disease.

Eat raspberries to reduce inflammation. They are a significant source of fiber, vitamin C, vitamin K, and manganese. Black raspberries are even more beneficial for reducing your risk of heart disease and high blood pressure.

Strawberries have a ton of vitamin C and protect against heart disease.

Grapes of any color are antioxidant powerhouses that reduce the risk of type 2 diabetes while also improving memory. They contain polyphenols that benefit your gut bacteria.

Goji berries, found in many Asian grocery stores, add minor amounts of iron to your diet.

How should you incorporate these foods into your diet? Put berries on a salad, in a bowl of yogurt, or on desserts and pastries. For a more savory experience, add them to pork, white fish, or chicken dishes.

Avocados

I've already mentioned that avocados are good for skin due to their high level of vitamin E. The beta carotene, protein, lecithin, fatty acids, vitamins A, and vitamin D in avocados are linked to skin membrane health, which helps moisturize your skin and protect it from damaging UV rays. This doesn't mean you can skip sunscreen if you eat avocados. These ingredients can also increase collagen metabolism and improve symptoms of psoriasis.

You've probably heard that avocados are a good source of "healthy fats." This is because they are monounsaturated oils that maintain healthy cholesterol levels and improve heart health.

Nuts

For a source of good fats, eat nuts. They contain protein, which is important for healthy bones, muscles, and skin. Remember, a reasonable amount of fat is beneficial for your skin. Nuts are also a healthy source of fiber.

Black walnuts and almonds are high in protein and low in saturated fats, although almonds are actually a seed that's grouped with nuts. Some nuts are heart healthy, including almonds (its skin has the highest concentration of antioxidants), hazelnuts, macadamia nuts, and pecans.

Because a serving of cashews (also technically a seed) contains 80% of your daily recommended dose of copper, they help prevent osteoporosis. Pistachios are lower in calories and fat than many other nuts, while also delivering protein, essential amino acids, fiber, and vitamins B1 and B6.

Fatty Fish

Fatty fish contains healthy fats, omega-3 fatty acids, vitamin E, protein, and zinc. Omega-3 fatty acids include EPA (eicosapentaenoic acid), DHA (docosahexaenoic acid), and ALA (alpha-linolenic acid), which are known for their anti-inflammatory properties. Studies have shown that omega-3 fats help reduce the pain of arthritis and are beneficial to those diagnosed with lupus. Vitamin E is one of the critical antioxidants for your skin and helps defend it against inflammation, like the inflammation associated with acne.

Healthy and sustainable fish sources include wild Alaskan salmon, wild Atlantic mackerel, wild-caught pacific (US) sardines, and farmed algae/seaweed. Sustainable sources change over time, but there are guides for sustainable sourcing.

Olive Oil

Olive oil is a food used internally and externally, meaning it is edible and topically applied to skin.

It's the oleic acid in olive oil, a type of fatty acid, that helps skin stay soft and smooth. Inflammatory processes often contribute to wrinkling and sagging, and oleic acid in olive oil reduces inflammation. Oleic acid is an antioxidant powerhouse, maintaining heart health, preventing diabetes, lowering blood pressure and cholesterol, preventing obesity, and protecting against cancer.

Oleic acid is found in foods other than olive oil, including beef, chicken, pork, sunflower seeds, eggs, pasta, olives, and milk.

Antioxidants

Why should you eat foods that contain antioxidants? Because antioxidants help your body fight off free radical damage. Free radicals are unstable molecules that steal electrons from other molecules, causing damage to DNA and other cells. Excess free radicals lead to certain diseases and speeds up aging. Antioxidants neutralize free radicals, preventing the damage they cause.

To some extent, controlling free radical damage slows skin aging. For example, living in a polluted area exposes you to extra free radical damage. It's possible to minimize the negative effects of free radicals by eating salmon, flaxseed (sprouted and ground), broccoli, cooked tomatoes, and almonds.

Foods containing antioxidants reduce fine lines, improve skin thickness, boost hydration, increase blood flow, and enhance skin texture. They also help slow the aging process by impairing harmful free radicals.

Foods that contain omega-3 fatty acids are excellent sources of antioxidants. Common antioxidants related to skin care include vitamins A, C, and E. Find vitamin A in liver, sweet potatoes, carrots, milk, and egg yolks. Vitamin C sources include oranges, black currants, kiwis, mangoes, strawberries, and spinach. Vitamin E is found in wheatgerm oil, avocados, nuts, seeds, and whole grains.

Water

Why mention water in a chapter about food? Well, Chinese medicine considers water an essential ingredient for healthy skin. Some in Chinese medicine even call the consumption of water an "art." Drink it at room temperature, not iced. Drink a glass first thing in the morning. Your cells need water to stay plump, and drinking water is an easy way to keep skin looking plump and moist.

Staying hydrated by drinking water and eating water-rich foods like cucumbers and watermelon further supports skin health by maintaining moisture balance. A nutritious, skin-friendly diet can enhance your natural glow and overall well-being.

Addressing Skin Issues
with Diet or Food

The link between diet and skin health is profound because the nutrients and substances in the food we consume significantly impact our skin's appearance, elasticity, and ability to heal. A well-balanced diet rich in vitamins, minerals, and antioxidants can promote a glowing complexion and reduce skin issues like acne, dryness, and premature aging.

As I've already discussed, antioxidants such as berries, leafy greens, and nuts combat oxidative stress and reduce inflammation, which can protect skin cells from damage caused by free radicals. Vitamin C-rich foods support collagen production, essential for maintaining skin elasticity and preventing wrinkles. Similarly, omega-3 fatty acids found in salmon, walnuts, and flaxseeds maintain skin hydration and reduce inflammation, which can ease conditions like eczema and psoriasis.

On the other hand, diets high in sugar and refined carbohydrates lead to glycation, a process where sugar molecules damage collagen and elastin, resulting in sagging and wrinkles. Excessive consumption of processed foods and trans fats can also exacerbate acne and inflammation. So, if you're experiencing a skin condition, first consider your diet. Here are a few issues and how you should eat to alleviate them.

Dark Circles

If you have dark circles under your eyes, the cause could be blood stagnation, a condition that peanuts help. Eat raw organic peanuts rather than those that are roasted in oil and salted. Eggplant is another food that reduces blood stagnation and swelling. Spinach, kale, and broccoli contain vitamin K, which boosts blood circulation of the skin and improves its texture.

Red Skin

Some people have redness or rosacea in their face. Sun damage sometimes results in broken capillaries that make the face look red. The skin appears much redder because the vessels are distended and filled with blood that no longer flows.

In TCM, excess heat in the body's system can also cause redness, such as overeating spicy food resulting in redder or drier skin.

One food that reduces heat (and therefore redness) is asparagus, which also detoxifies and promotes blood circulation. Promoting blood circulation in the skin is key to maintaining its integrity and suppleness. Carrots and mung beans also detoxify while they clear heat.

Sun damage reduces suppleness (or softness) in the skin. This is because of the drying heat that makes the skin hard, not flexible. White rice not only clears heat but also builds yin (the fluid part of the yin-yang pairing). Other foods that clear heat are bok choy, red and green cabbage, cucumbers, bananas, celery, peaches, pineapple, lentils, sweet potatoes, cantaloupe, and figs.

Acne

I previously mentioned foods that detoxify. Why bring it up again? Because acne and some other skin conditions are, in part, because of your body's attempt to rid itself of toxins. Eating foods that naturally and gently detoxify your body leads to clearer and more healthy skin.

The list of foods that detoxify includes pumpkin seeds, sunflower seeds, soybeans, olives, and rice vinegar. Shiitake mushrooms and tea also promote digestion, and a digestive system that works well definitely reflects in your skin.

In modern medicine, green tea is a super antioxidant (anti-ager) and in Chinese medicine, a super detoxifier. It contains flavonoids, vitamin C, vitamin E, carotene, and much more. Green tea helps protect your skin from sun damage, secondhand tobacco smoke, and stress.

Speaking of toxic heat causing acne, processed foods are the bane of your skin's existence. Most are processed using high heat, and that heat transfers into your body and skin. Try your best to avoid eating too many processed foods. Chemically processed foods contain high levels of sodium, sugar, and fat, leading to obesity, type 2 diabetes, heart disease, and other chronic health conditions. Our government mandates nutritional information on labels, but frankly, many people don't read labels or *know* how much daily sodium intake is unhealthy.

Almost all processed foods are ground up and pasteurized, which doesn't lessen the healthfulness of the food, but chemically processed foods are different because of the added sugars, fats, salts, and artificial ingredients. More sugar means no essential nutrients, more calories, and potentially more acne. When our body gets overloaded with sugar, it detoxes via acne. Trans fats increase inflammation in the body, which is the source of many symptoms and can lead to higher cholesterol and more acne (inflammation). Furthermore, highly processed foods are usually low in fiber, which is important for gut health and heart health.

Dr. Joel Fuhrman has written about what he calls "Fast Food Genocide." In his articles, he discusses the negative effects processed foods have on mental and emotional health if you're interested in reading more about processed food.

Moisture and Elasticity of Skin

Our skin is nourished by blood flow; therefore, it makes sense to eat foods that nourish blood. Again, this is a way for you to maintain your vibrant appearance and strengthen anti-aging treatments.

Red beets are a blood nourishing food, and they also calm your spirit. Ah, a calming food. Don't like canned beets? Steamed or baked fresh beets are delicious. If you don't want to eat them plain (but take my word for it; they are yummy!) then put them in a salad. Add some mixed greens, goat cheese, nuts, and pears or apples with the beets. It's a great lunch or dinner salad.

Eggs not only tonify blood, but they also nourish yin (the moistening part of the yin/yang pair) to keep your skin moist. This category of foods is important for anyone who is interested in having vibrant looking skin. Walnuts are a time-honored food in Chinese medicine for nourishing the skin. They contain anti-aging substances like linolenic and oleic acids, carotene, and vitamins B1 and B2.

Essential fatty acids keep cell walls strong to retain moisture, helping your skin look plump and refreshed. The best sources of essential fatty acids are salmon, sardines, tuna, avocados, nuts, and seeds.

Protein enhances skin elasticity because fibroblasts, which produce collagen and elastin, rely on protein for their formation. Boost your protein intake with sources such as meat, eggs, cheese, milk, yogurt, beans, and nuts.

Digestive Health

Digestion is not only important for general health but for your skin as well. You may have noticed that I talk a lot about proper digestion. According to Chinese medicine, when your digestion works properly, it reflects in your skin because it allows blood to nourish your skin. Food feeds your skin, especially when you eat consciously. While you eat, don't drive, don't talk on the phone, don't work on your laptop, etc. The point? Eating well is something that is imperative for good health; therefore, it deserves your full attention. When you are active while eating, you miss the pleasure of eating. If you're not paying attention, you may not chew your food enough, which means you aren't absorbing all the nutritional value from the food. Many of the important nutrients in foods are released and made more available after food is completely chewed. When you eat fast and don't chew completely, you also misjudge the quantity of the food you eat, leading to weight gain issues.

Food spends two to four hours inside our stomach, so theoretically we shouldn't be hungry for those hours. It's a matter of eating slowly enough that your brain receives the "I'm full" signal from your stomach. If you eat too quickly, you are more likely to overeat before your brain registers as satisfied. Putting your fork down between bites slows down your eating.

Foods That Promote Digestion

Here are some foods that assist with digestion in a way that will reflect in your skin: Anise seed, turbinado sugar, cinnamon, fennel seed, and molasses.

Ginger is a powerful herb in Chinese medicine because it aids digestion. It is used to treat morning sickness and other types of nausea.

Yogurt includes friendly bacteria that help your gut stay balanced. Kefir is a probiotic yogurt drink also filled with good bacteria.

Sourdough bread is made with fermented dough and is easier to digest than white bread. Its energy releases more slowly so it keeps your blood sugar managed.

Fatty acids and polyphenols, found in olive oil, reduce gut inflammation and indigestion, and they improve pancreas health.

Eat vegetables and fruits because gut bacteria need fiber to flourish.

Cherries beautify the skin through digestion, and they are rich in iron, so they enrich blood flow to your skin.

Eating Habits

Eat Organic

Eat organic when it's available, especially meat, dairy, and foods like apples that are eaten in their entirety. Understand that the nutritional value of many organically grown and raised foods is the same as conventionally grown foods. The difference is that organic foods are grown with fewer synthetic pesticides, fertilizers, hormones, and antibiotics. Some organic foods have different nutritional values, like organic meats and dairy. And eggs have higher levels of omega-3 fatty acids, which are more heart-healthy than other fats. The USDA has a certification program that requires organic food growers to meet strict government standards, so you can trust the USDA Organic label.

Eat Larger Meals Earlier

An important saying to remember is, "Eat like an emperor in the morning, like a prince at midday, and like a pauper in the evening." According to Chinese medicine, our digestive system is at its highest energetic activity early in the day. When you eat at night, your digestion isn't as capable of digesting food as it is in the morning. And the energy created from dinner is wasted because you're going to bed in just a few hours. Plus, eating late in the evening is associated with weight gain and/or obesity. Better to boost your energy in the morning and afternoon from healthy, slightly larger meals. Plus, you'll be less hungry in the evening and less likely to eat a large meal if you eat well earlier.

Warm Not Cold

In Chinese medicine, sweet foods have a warm energy, and our digestive system loves warmth. Don't overeat sweets; everything in moderation. If you want your digestion to work smoothly, no iced drinks please. Iced drinks and foods that have a cold energy stress your digestive system. Consuming cold food and drinks and making your digestion work hard to warm up the food makes your digestion sluggish or leads to food retention, which will make you feel bloated. If you stress your digestion, help it with bamboo shoots and bell peppers. Plums, tomatoes, oats, and peas also harmonize digestion. And parsley isn't just a garnish; it enhances your digestive system.

Good digestion is important for your general health and for radiant skin. Your skin reflects your general health and how well your digestion works: the inside reflects on the outside. If you feel like your digestion needs improvement, see a practitioner of Chinese medicine who will improve your health with acupuncture and provide nutritional advice. Chinese medicine has an entire arm of nutrition for improving health.

Good digestion goes hand in hand with healthy, youthful skin. I know it sounds trite, but "you are what you eat." What we put into our bodies affects how we look on the outside. Now go start your new and improved grocery list.

SUPPLEMENTS

CHAPTER 5

It's paradoxical that the idea of living a long life appeals to everyone but the idea of getting old doesn't appeal to anyone.

- Andy Rooney

WE CAN'T AVOID aging because it is inevitable. Yet most of us want to hold on to our youthfulness as long as we can. The best way to promote longevity and to feel good while the years pass is to take good care of your body. You do that by eating nutritious foods, moving your body, getting regular exercise, skipping smoking, managing stress, and taking vitamins and supplements. These include vitamins A through D, calcium, CoQ10, alpha-linolenic acid, among others. Some supplements not only support healthy aging but also slow certain aging processes.

The Role of Supplements in Aging Well

Vitamin A

Vitamin A is fat-soluble and a powerful antioxidant that is an integral part of maintaining overall good health and your skin's integrity. Vitamin A keeps skin healthy and plays a role in immune system functioning, proper growth, bone formation, reproduction, and wound healing. Symptoms of vitamin A deficiency include dry eyes, night blindness, diarrhea, and skin problems. Vitamin A comes from retinoids found in animal sources and carotenoids in plants. Retinol is the purest form of vitamin A, and it's recommended for use in your skin care routine. The carotenoid form acts as an antioxidant in the body, has cancer-fighting properties, and is an anti-inflammatory. Research shows that people who eat foods rich in vitamin A maintain good vision longer and are less likely to develop both cataracts and age-related macular degeneration.

I have heard vitamin A called a "wonder vitamin" for the skin. Whether eating A in food, taking it in a supplement, or using it topically in your skin care products, it does the following:

- Slows signs of skin aging
- Encourages skin cell production
- Smooths wrinkles
- Evens skin tone
- Clears acne
- Gives skin a healthy glow

Adequate amounts of vitamin A are required for the development of epithelial cells, which are among the most abundant cells in the skin's outermost layers. This is where skin regenerates and helps prevent acne and wrinkles.

In the retinyl form, it's found in beef, calf, and chicken liver, eggs, fish liver oils, whole milk, whole milk yogurt, cottage cheese, butter, and cheeses. Food sources of the carotenoid form of vitamin A include sweet potatoes, yams, cantaloupe, kale, turnip greens, collard greens, cilantro, fresh thyme, broccoli, apricots, asparagus, beets, spinach, carrots, and butternut squash.

The B Vitamins

The B vitamins are integral in the formation of every cell in your body. They are often grouped together as vitamin B complex because many have similar properties, are in the same natural sources, and their physiological functions overlap. Each B vitamin is important for your metabolism and digestion, breaking down food and turning it into energy. That's why feeling tired or fatigued is a sign of vitamin B deficiency. Taking a B complex supplement is one way to absorb the correct amount of each B vitamin.

Here are reasons each of the B vitamins is important to maintain overall good health, digestion, and vibrant skin.

B1 (Thiamine)

Vitamin B1 or thiamine is named "B1" because it was the first B vitamin discovered. It is called the "anti-stress vitamin" because it improves the body's ability to withstand stressful circumstances, partly by strengthening the immune system. Three other functions include changing carbohydrates into energy, playing a role in nerve conduction, and helping to fight depression.

Symptoms of low levels of B1 include fatigue, irritability, nerve damage, sleep disturbances, loss of appetite, digestive distress, and poor memory.

Vitamin B1 alleviates red, irritated, acne-prone skin. It also improves the appearance of fine lines and wrinkles by preventing oxidation that causes free radicals that damage healthy skin's basic building blocks. The breakdown of the skin is one cause of wrinkles, thinner skin, and dull skin.

Food sources for B1 include enriched white rice or egg noodles, fortified cereals, whole grains, corn, seafood, pork, sunflower seeds, acorn squash, and black beans.

B2 (Riboflavin)

B2 or riboflavin works as an antioxidant and metabolizes carbohydrates, fats, and protein into glucose to boost energy. It aids in maintaining a healthy digestive system and a strong immune system. Having adequate amounts of it in your system fosters healthy skin and hair. Riboflavin is necessary for normal development, physical performance, lactation, and reproduction. Vitamin B6 is activated by riboflavin, which is another example of how the B vitamins work synergistically.

Vitamin B2 improves skin tone, reduces inflammation, and balances skin's natural oils, making it effective against both dry skin and acne. It does this by aiding cell turnover and collagen maintenance, both of which protect the skin's integrity.

Anemia, cataracts, fatigue, migraines, night blindness, and red itchy eyes are signs of vitamin B2 deficiency. According to the NIH, though vitamin B2 deficiency is not frequently seen in the United States, people who are more likely to have a deficiency are alcoholics, women on birth control pills, and older adults.

Food sources for riboflavin include whole grains, almonds, wild rice, mushrooms, eggs, broccoli, dairy products, soybeans, brewer's yeast, and spinach.

B3 (Niacin)

Vitamin B3 is also known as niacinamide and nicotinic acid. All tissues in the body use it for basic metabolic processes. Like B2, it is involved in the transformation of carbohydrates, fats, and proteins into energy. Studies show that nicotinic acid is effective in raising HDL (good) cholesterol levels while reducing LDL (bad) cholesterol and triglyceride levels, which reduces the risk of cardiovascular disease.

B3 prevents water loss, so skin better retains moisture, reducing the appearance of wrinkles. Topically, it reduces hyperpigmentation (age spots), melasma, and redness because of its anti-inflammatory properties. Studies show that it also improves the elasticity of the skin.

Vitamin B3 is found in fish (salmon, tuna), chicken, lean red meat, brown and white rice, peanuts, sunflower seeds, whole wheat bread, bananas, broccoli, tofu, milk, and eggs.

B5 (Pantothenic Acid)

B5 or pantothenic acid is involved in a variety of the body's metabolic processes, including energy generation, like the other B vitamins. It also works in the synthesis of hormones. Headaches, fatigue, numbness, and muscle cramps are signs of vitamin B5 deficiency.

As part of its role in our metabolism, B5 maintains optimal conditions for good skin, hair, and nails. It acts as a moisturizer and enhances the healing process of the skin, reducing issues such as acne breakouts. Dermatologists also use it in cream form to treat atopic dermatitis.

It is found in a variety of plant and animal foods, including beef, chicken, seafood, avocados, mushrooms, potatoes, peanuts, sunflower seeds, milk, yogurt, broccoli, and eggs, to name a few.

B6 (Pyridoxine, Pyridoxal, Pyridoxamine)

Vitamin B6 is involved in enzyme and protein metabolism and the biosynthesis of neurotransmitters.

B6 or pyridoxine eases hormonal imbalances that lead to wrinkles and acne breakouts. Having a B6 deficiency is associated with dermatitis.

It is found in foods that include salmon, tuna, beef liver and other organ meats, poultry, cottage cheese, turkey, dark leafy greens, onions, spinach, and tuna.

B7 (Biotin)

B7 or biotin is commonly used to treat skin, hair, and nail conditions that include rashes, hair loss, and brittle nails. It evens out skin, plays a role in maintaining plump, hydrated skin, and revitalizes dull, aging skin. It is required for healthy cell growth and repair.

Food sources include protein-rich foods, grains, nuts, egg yolks, salmon, apples, sweet potatoes, tuna, spinach, broccoli, cheddar cheese, milk, oatmeal, and pork.

B9 (Folic Acid)

Folic acid (B9) makes DNA and other genetic materials in the body. That means it is an important supplement for women who may get pregnant or who are pregnant because adequate amounts of folic acid prevents neural tube defects.

B9 or folic acid increases hydration by maintaining skin's barrier function. This helps ease dryness and maintains adequate collagen production. Folic acid supplementation is used to treat psoriasis.

Eat nuts, whole wheat bread, dark green leafy vegetables (spinach, turnip greens), fresh fruits, whole grains, and seafood to absorb a supply of B9.

B12 (Cobalamin)

Vitamin B12 regulates digestion, energy metabolism, mood, sleep, weight, and fertility. It also reduces brain fog or memory issues and prevents anemia. It keeps your body's nerve cells healthy and is a part of the DNA process of every cell.

Regarding your skin, B12 or cobalamin reduces inflammation, dryness, and acne. It also lessens the appearance of psoriasis, dermatitis, hyperpigmentation, and eczema.

Good sources of B12 include eggs, meat, fish, milk and milk products, clams, oysters, and fortified cereals.

B-Complex

As you may have gathered from this section, many of the B vitamins work synergistically and have similar functions. It makes sense to prepare them as a complex. A B-complex vitamin supplement reduces fatigue as well as improves mood and cognitive performance. B vitamins produce the neurotransmitters serotonin, dopamine, and norepinephrine, which explains why people feel less moody after taking B complex. The vitamins in the complex form also convert carbohydrates into ATP to help muscles create and store energy. B-complex supports our physical body, nervous system, and emotional self.

Whew! There's a lot of information to keep track of regarding B vitamins. Consider an injection of Bs to benefit your skin, memory, digestion, and metabolism.

Vitamin C (Ascorbic Acid)

Vitamin C or ascorbic acid is essential for a healthy immune system. Our adrenal glands need vitamin C to synthesize adrenaline for energy and increase dopamine to regulate moods. It's also critical for the strength of bones, muscles, and tendons, and is needed to reduce fatigue and muscle pain. People with vitamin C deficiency are often fatigued and depressed. A severe deficiency is a cause of scurvy, which is a fatal disease not heard about much these days. Humans are the only animals whose bodies can't make vitamin C so we must absorb it from foods or supplements.

Vitamin C is good for the skin because it stimulates collagen growth and production, helping us look younger. Adding vitamin C to cultures of skin fibroblasts leads to the production of collagen according to research. Because it's an antioxidant and is an integral part of our cell matrix, vitamin C is especially important for the skin as collagen and elastin are a part of the cellular matrix. Collagen and elastin are especially vulnerable to free radical damage, and adequate levels of vitamin C prevent damage.

In addition, vitamin C assists the antioxidant power of vitamin E when used together. It protects the skin from UV ray damage through its antioxidant properties. Our bodies lack the enzyme necessary to convert glucose to ascorbic acid, so we must eat foods rich in vitamin C or take supplements. Using products with both vitamin C and vitamin E increases UV protection of skin cells as compared to using each on its own.

Increased concentration of vitamin C in the skin—either topically or through a supplement—protects the skin from free radical damage. But researchers recommend applying it topically for the best results. Studies conducted on half a face showed reduced wrinkles, increased collagen and firmness, improved skin tone and pigmentation, and decreased roughness on the side of the face treated with a serum containing vitamin C. One study even reported a decrease in deep furrows.

Food sources of vitamin C include citrus fruits, berries, peas, green leafy vegetables, broccoli, kale, and turnip greens. If you take a supplement, take it daily because of its water solubility.

Calcium

Calcium is the most abundant mineral in the body and plays a critical role in numerous bodily functions. It is essential for building and maintaining strong bones and teeth, which store about 99% of the body's calcium. Beyond bone health, calcium is crucial for muscle contraction, nerve transmission, and blood clotting. It also helps regulate heart rhythms and supports the release of hormones and enzymes that aid various metabolic processes.

A low level of calcium causes extreme fatigue, insomnia, and brain fog. Low levels are also associated with anxiety and a negative mood. A higher calcium level is associated with protective effects on mental health. An adequate amount of calcium is an important part of cellular energy production and keeps the metabolism working well and level. Proper levels of calcium are associated with lower perceived stress, lower anxiety scores, and higher positive mood and resilience scores. It's also a significant factor in REM sleep because it helps our body use the amino acid tryptophan, which leads to relaxation. These results are, in part, because calcium regulates neurotransmitter synthesis, which plays an important role in mood regulation.

When exposed to sunlight, skin produces vitamin D, which is necessary for the proper absorption of calcium. Necessary calcium content in the epidermis maintains skin's barrier, repair, and self-replenishing functions. Stress, not enough sleep, and feeling anxious leads to skin looking dull, while calcium preserves hydration and a healthy skin glow.

For women, being in or nearing menopause may be the beginning of bone loss or osteoporosis. Combine calcium and vitamin D for optimal bone health and to prevent bone loss and reduce the risk of fractures.

We all know there is calcium in milk, and some companies fortify cereals and juices with calcium. Other food sources include cheese and yogurt, dark leafy green vegetables, almonds, tofu, and sardines.

IMPORTANT FACT
Our bodies only metabolize 500 mg of calcium at a time so split doses to include 500 mg three times a day. Otherwise, you excrete what you don't absorb.

Vitamin D (The Sunshine Vitamin)

Your body naturally produces vitamin D when your skin is exposed to sunlight. Skin becomes drier when the body is deficient in vitamin D and there is an increased risk of conditions like psoriasis. Because people may spend more time inside, especially during very hot and cold weather, they can become deficient in vitamin D. We also absorb less D from the sun while wearing sunscreen. Therefore, supplements are usually recommended.

Vitamin D sources include milk fortified with vitamin D, herring, broccoli, figs, oats, and salmon. According to recommendations from the National Institutes of Health Consensus Conference on Osteoporosis, once a woman has reached perimenopause, she should take 1500 mg/day of calcium fortified with 200 to 400 IU of vitamin D. Doing so will contribute to a healthier menopause experience through improved vaginal and genitourinary health, as well as bone density.

Vitamin E

Vitamin E is a fat-soluble vitamin with several forms and functions. Alpha-tocopherol is the most active form of vitamin E and a powerful biological antioxidant. It works to maintain cell integrity, protect our cells against the effects of free radicals, and has shown to play a role in DNA repair. For couples who are trying to get pregnant, it increases cervical mucus in women, allowing sperm to live longer. It enhances the overall efficiency of male reproductive systems too.

Vitamin E is important for healthy vision, skin, and brain function. A deficiency in vitamin E can contribute to depressive symptoms, and studies show it plays a role in modulating major depressive disorder. It is an anti-inflammatory and anti-cancer, and it's important for maintaining a healthy central nervous system. It also helps the body produce enough red blood cells to prevent fatigue and supports the regulation of cholesterol levels. Take vitamin E if you're feeling tired, have a low sex drive, are susceptible to colds, suffer from allergies, or experience mild depression.

Your skin's natural oils include vitamin E, so adding more of it stops your skin from losing moisture. As an antioxidant and anti-inflammatory, vitamin E minimizes your skin's aging process. Antioxidants prevent free radicals from damaging molecules and DNA. Vitamin E oil is very beneficial to your skin. It moisturizes, nourishes, reduces hyperpigmentation, and decreases wrinkling.

What foods contain vitamin E? Try vegetable oils, nuts, green leafy vegetables, egg yolks, wheat germ oil, spinach, kiwis, and mangoes.

Lipids

Lipids include fats and lecithin, and they play an essential role in maintaining healthy, smooth skin, especially in the stratum corneum. And cells require lipids for damage repair. More and more attention is being paid to the use of lipids for skin care because they form a protective barrier, preventing moisture loss and protecting against environmental damage.

Eating a proper balance of omega-3 and omega-6 fats improves skin. I advise many of my patients to take both fish oil and flaxseed oil. Lipids are in milk, egg yolks, soybeans, canola oil, wheat germ, and corn.

Alpha-Linolenic Acid

Alpha-linolenic acid (ALA) is an essential fatty acid in the omega family. It acts as an antioxidant that helps regulate skin moisture and nutrient absorption while providing protection against environmental damage. ALA, a vital omega-3 fatty acid, helps maintain the skin's natural barrier, reducing moisture loss and protecting against dryness. It also has anti-inflammatory properties, soothing irritated or sensitive skin and aiding in conditions like eczema or acne. Additionally, it promotes collagen production, enhancing skin elasticity and reducing signs of aging. Regular intake of ALA through diet or skin care helps achieve smooth, hydrated, and resilient skin.

A small amount of it is found in leafy green vegetables, but the best way to get it is by eating ground flaxseed. Other foods containing it are canola oil, safflower oil, sunflower oil, corn oil, hemp oil, wheat germ, pumpkin, soybeans, walnuts, salmon, and mackerel.

Minerals

Vitamins and minerals are essential for the effective functioning of the cells and organs in our body. Skin is the largest living organ in the body, so use minerals to stay healthy and vibrant. Two of the most important and well researched are copper and selenium.

Copper, in conjunction with vitamin C and zinc, develops elastin. In one wrinkle study, participants who used copper-rich cream reported rapid changes, such as overall skin improvement and reduction of fine lines and wrinkles.

The Journal of the American Medical Association (JAMA) reported that selenium plays a key role in the prevention of skin cancer. Selenium is found in seafood and eggs. However, taking selenium does not mean that you can sunbathe. Once again, I will remind you to protect your skin from the sun with sunscreen.

Supplements

I recommend certain supplements to my patients. It's just nearly impossible to get all the nutrients we need from food these days. There are all kinds of obstacles in our way. Soil has become depleted of vitamins and minerals. We live active lives and lack time to prepare the food necessary for good health. Many of us can't follow the seasons and eat only food grown in our region because our growing seasons are too short. So, for most of us, it makes sense to take high-quality supplements.

Take careful consideration when choosing supplements. Buy supplements that are tested to ensure they contain the ingredients listed on the label and are free from harmful contaminants. An organization like USP or Consumer Lab may certify them.

Scrutinize the ingredient list on supplement bottles. Avoid any with unnecessary additives, fillers, or artificial colors. These substances offer no nutritional benefit and can cause adverse reactions in some people. You can also look at the brand's reputation. Look for companies that prioritize transparency and provide detailed information about sourcing, manufacturing, and ingredient origins.

Consult healthcare professionals before starting any new supplement. They can help you determine what you really need based on your health needs. This is especially true in Chinese medicine because nutritional supplements can contain herbal ingredients as well.

Choosing the Right Supplements

To ensure you choose the right supplements for healthy skin, start by identifying your skin's needs, such as dryness, acne, aging, or sensitivity. This helps target the most beneficial supplements for you.

Key nutrients to look for include antioxidants like vitamin C and E, which combat free radicals and boost collagen production. Omega-3 fatty acids, found in fish oil or flaxseed oil supplements, promote hydration and reduce inflammation. Collagen peptides can improve skin elasticity and minimize wrinkles, while biotin supports overall skin health.

Consider supplements with zinc or probiotics if acne or skin inflammation is a concern because they regulate sebum production and support a healthy gut-skin axis. Hyaluronic acid supplements enhance skin hydration from within, ideal for combating dryness.

Before starting any supplement, consult a dermatologist or healthcare provider, especially if you have underlying health conditions or take medications. Ensure the supplements are high quality by checking for third-party testing and reputable brands.

Always remember that supplements work best when combined with a balanced diet, hydration, proper skin care, and sun protection. They are not a substitute for a healthy lifestyle, but they can complement your overall skin routine effectively.

WEIGHT

CHAPTER 6

One day you will look back and see that all
along you were blooming.

- Morgan Harper Nichols

W<small>E HAVE ALL</small> received the message about a healthy weight being associated with a lower risk for many diseases and health issues. Keeping weight steady over time lowers the risk for heart disease, many cancers, hypertension (high blood pressure), gallstones, sleep apnea, stroke, and diabetes, to name a few. There is a strong negative effect of obesity on longevity, making it a topic of particular interest regarding healthy aging.

Obesity is a multifactor chronic disease that is caused by a variety of influences, and those same variables differ from person to person. It involves excessive deposits of white fat in the body and reduces metabolic fitness. Healthy weight depends on age, sex, body frame, genetics, etc., meaning everyone has their own healthy numbers. What *your* healthy weight is and what causes *you* to gain or lose weight differs from what affects someone else's weight gain or loss.

Bottom line, it is best for overall general health not to be overweight or underweight. Both are associated with negative health outcomes, but obesity is much more prevalent regarding poor aging. A simplistic explanation is "energy in, energy out." "Energy in" comes from the food and drink we consume. "Energy out" is the energy/calories we use to live: breathing, digesting, and other physical activities. Too much energy in and not enough out leads to weight gain. More energy out than taken in eventually leads to weight loss.

Obesity also changes the physiology of the skin in terms of mechanical friction, skin infections and irritations, skin tags, dryness, and even melanoma. In Chinese medicine, we talk about the skin reflecting what is happening internally: the outside reflects the inside. So, when changes in hormones, growth factors, and fat cells occur on the inside, it affects the way your skin looks.

The skin may stretch as a person grows heavier. In severe cases of obesity, the skin can become less sensitized to pain because of poor vascularization. There's just too much flesh for the blood vessels to serve. Other issues include impaired collagen production and impaired lymphatic flow that leads to swelling and puffiness. Your skin becomes thicker and oilier, causing skin folds and irritating breakouts. Obesity aggravates psoriasis, and cellulite, a normal, age-related dimpling of the skin, becomes more pronounced.

I can't speak to what is a healthy weight for you specifically. Check statistics on height and BMI. Also talk with your doctor. There's obesity, there's being too skinny, and there's somewhere in the middle. Find the place in the middle that feels good for you.

Factors Influencing Weight and Aging

There are several factors associated with your ability to live a healthy-weight lifestyle.

Genetics

Although lifestyle is a key driving factor for obesity, some people are genetically predisposed to gain or retain extra weight around their middle. However, genetics doesn't perfectly explain the heritability of obesity. For example, about 50% of overweight children carry extra pounds into adulthood. While chromosomal abnormalities play a part, maternal nutrition during pregnancy, exposure to toxins, high levels of stress, and general overall health of the mother are all relevant factors.

People are *not* destined to be overweight because of genetics. Obesity results from the interaction between environmental and innate or genetic factors. Studies recommend lifestyle habits like eating a healthy diet, staying active/exercising, and avoiding unhealthy habits to overcome a genetic tendency toward being overweight.

Diet and Nutrition

I dislike the word *diet*. THIS IS IMPORTANT. It's not about dieting, it's about lifestyle. In fact, the origin of the word *diet* is from the Greek *diaita*, which means "a way of life" or "regimen." There it is: lifestyle! The word has such a negative connotation now—restricting types and amounts of food. You can't eat this, you can't eat that, no dessert, etc. And when will my diet be over? This is the thing that most people want to know: how long will

I be on this diet? Stop it! It's about deciding to reach a healthy weight and changing your lifestyle. It's a forever thing to achieve a weight that feels comfortable and healthy. It's the weight that makes you love your body and stay there because you have a new, healthy lifestyle.

Many programs are available, including family healthy weight programs, food service and nutrition guidelines, diabetes prevention programs, and more. Check with the government and other organizations for a list of specific programs. Whatever program you choose, you can embrace a new life with:

- Fresher approach to eating
- Renewed perspective on food and its role in your life
- Deeper love and appreciation for yourself
- Restored joy and enthusiasm for exercise
- Better ability to make mindful and enjoyable food choices
- Healthier ways to cope with stress
- Stronger willpower to handle cravings

… all leading to a vibrant, fulfilling new life.

Most weight loss programs, be it a program, plan, or prescription, do *not* actually result in weight loss. That's because having a healthy weight is a lifestyle, not a diet.

Stress and Environment

The main issue with stress is that it leads to unhealthy eating habits. Some people "stress eat." Eating, especially eating fat, warms up the body and gives a person a sense of comfort. That's why it's called "comfort food." Stress elevates cortisol in the body, causing cravings for unhealthy foods like highly processed snacks or high sugar sweets. The cortisol spike also kills your motivation to prepare a healthy meal.

A review in PubMed highlights several ways stress can lead to weight gain and negatively impact the skin:

- **Reduced Activity Levels**: Stress often disrupts daily routines and lowers physical activity, leading to a more sedentary lifestyle.

- **Decreased Self-Regulation**: Stress reduces our ability to make healthy choices, leading to bad eating habits. Consuming excess sugar and fat can lead to skin problems, such as increased breakouts.

- **Sleep Disruption**: Stress can interfere with sleep quality and duration. Sleep deprivation is directly linked to weight gain and obesity. Poor bedtime habits, often caused by stress, exacerbate the issue, resulting in dull, lifeless skin.

- **Hormonal Changes**: Stress alters hormone levels, increasing stress-related eating and stimulating cravings. These hormonal shifts can mimic the effects of life changes like perimenopause, causing drier skin, increased breakouts, and formation of wrinkles.

Proper stress management is essential not just for maintaining a healthy weight but also for ensuring vibrant, healthy skin.

Meditation

To manage stress, mindfulness is one of the most studied strategies. The concept is based on Buddhism. Focus on your experience at the moment without judgment. It's about processing the sensations of the moment using breathing techniques, body scanning, meditation, and gentle movement. Focusing on the present moment reduces emotional stress and heart rate, leading to a calm experience. The process releases hormones and calms active and stressed parts of the brain. The resulting physiological changes allow one to be in stressful moments (since we all have them) but also cope with a skillful response rather than just automatically reacting with worry, fear, or sadness. It is a learned skill that improves general health, reduces symptoms like pain, and lowers anxiety and depression. No special equipment is required for most meditation techniques.

Physical Activity

While activity is important, I tell patients seeking weight loss that they can't run away from their fork. What do I mean by this? A person cannot exercise their way into a thinner body. That being said, exercise is important for achieving and maintaining a healthy weight.

It is important to find a type of exercise you enjoy enough to make time in your schedule to do it. Running is not suitable for everyone nor necessary. If you enjoy running, you don't have to be a marathon runner. Walking is a great exercise. Fifty years ago, *Prevention Magazine* published multiple articles about the health benefits of walking, and we still read about it today. Swimming, biking, yoga, and dance are other low-impact exercise choices. Whatever type of exercise you choose, schedule time to do it. For me, I love running at midday, so I don't see patients when it's time to run. Figure out what time of day is best for your self-care and do it.

Not only will your body and your general health thank you for exercising, so will your skin. Your skin has lots of blood vessels near the surface and when you exercise, you pump blood through these vessels, giving your skin a healthy glow. Exercise boosts collagen production, which helps your skin be more supple and prevents lines and wrinkles. This is because the increased blood flow brings nutrients to the fibroblasts that produce collagen and elastin.

Sleep

Studies show a relationship between sleep and weight. Sleep disruption leads to feeling tired, which leads us to drink more caffeine (a sleep disruptor) and eat high-calorie, sugary snacks. Both adults and children who cannot sleep weigh more than those who sleep normally. Sleep deprivation also makes our skin look dull … we just look tired.

Lack of sleep is one factor that leads to weight gain because of an increase in ghrelin, a hunger hormone. At the same time (double whammy), it reduces leptin, the satiation (I'm full) hormone. This leads to craving high-energy, high-calorie foods that are salty and sweet. Being tired and more emotional may also lead to stress-related eating or making poor decisions about food all around.

There are several common methods for improving sleep quality. Follow a sleep routine before bed: lower bright lights and leave your phone in another room. Make your bedroom a pleasant place for relaxation so that entering the room induces a calm feeling. Are you achy in the morning? You may need a new mattress. If you take naps during the day but can't seem to sleep well at night, then give up the naps. Don't drink caffeine within 6 hours of bedtime. Getting regular exercise positively affects sleep, but do it during the day, not right before bed. Do you usually need an alarm clock to wake up? Try waking up naturally to better understand your sleep patterns.

Weight Management Strategies for Anti-aging

Reducing Sodium Intake

For help to lose weight, consume 1,500 mg or less of sodium per day. While it may seem like a significant adjustment, this step enhances the effectiveness of any new eating plan. Begin by journaling your sodium intake for a week, noting which foods contribute the most sodium. The high sodium levels in many common foods may surprise you. For most people, cutting back on sodium is essential.

Excess sodium intake negatively affects your overall health. It contributes to high blood pressure, fluid retention (edema), weight gain, sleep disturbances, and even an increased risk of eczema (atopic dermatitis). If you notice puffiness on your face or body, excessive sodium consumption could be the culprit. In my cosmetic acupuncture courses, I often advise students to observe how salt affects their skin: eating a salty meal close to bedtime often results in puffy eyes by morning. Sodium dehydrates your skin, reducing its elasticity and making it prone to wrinkles.

Reducing sodium might sound simple, but it requires a conscious effort. The most effective approach is to avoid salty foods and minimize added salt in cooking and at the table. Sweating, crying, and urination all help eliminate sodium from the body. Staying well-hydrated is always a good practice, as it supports these natural processes and promotes overall health.

Reducing Saturated and Trans Fats

The second crucial weight loss advice I give to patients is to limit saturated fat intake to 15 grams or less per day. This isn't a permanent restriction, but achieving a leaner body (15-20% body fat) often requires reducing saturated fat and eliminating trans fats entirely.

Read labels. Again, just like decreasing sodium, it's surprising how many foods contain lots and lots of saturated fat. It's not only chocolate candy and ice cream, believe me.

Your body needs fat, but too much fat builds up cholesterol and may lead to conditions like heart disease and stroke. Saturated fats raise your bad (LDL) cholesterol and are often stored as visceral fat around your abdomen, contributing to weight gain.

To simplify this process for my patients, I recommend starting with a food journal. Record food content on your appointment calendar or use an app to track sodium and saturated fat grams consumed. Spend a week observing your habits and identifying high-fat foods in your diet. This is also a good time to begin a regular weight-check routine.

Incorporate healthier eating habits by adding more fruits and vegetables to your meals. Opt for fish, chicken, and lean cuts of meat, and avoid frying food. Switch to reduced-fat or fat-free dairy products. These changes not only support weight loss but also contribute to long-term health.

Hydration and Weight Loss

Drinking two glasses of water before meals helps people lose weight and keep it off. Water creates a feeling of fullness, leading to reduced calorie intake. It's an interesting fact that thirst masquerades as hunger and can lead to overeating. Staying hydrated not only curbs unnecessary snacking but also supports overall health.

As a runner, hydration is especially important to me, and I've often wondered what's best to drink before or after exercise: water, sports drinks like Gatorade, or even milk. A sign I recently saw claimed, "Milk hydrates better than water," which piqued my curiosity. After some research, I discovered that low-fat milk does indeed hydrate more effectively than water. It makes sense because milk contains nutrients like electrolytes, protein, and minerals, which both nourish and hydrate the body. Whole milk came in a close second to low-fat milk as a long-lasting hydration tool. Yes, milk is a hydration tool!

Water not only suppresses your appetite; it boosts your metabolism and makes exercising easier and more efficient. Proper hydration also reduces joint discomfort, making movement easier and more efficient. Your body needs water to burn fat! Dehydration causes brain fog, fatigue, dizziness, and lack of motivation.

What does water do for your skin? Make it look brighter. Research shows that increasing water intake is like applying a topical moisturizer. This means that water supports your skin's physiology, improving elasticity and preventing lines and wrinkles from forming. Whether you're aiming for better health, enhanced physical performance, or glowing skin, hydration is a fundamental step to achieving your goals.

Cutting Calories

When you consume calories, your body either uses them for energy or stores them as fat, creating a "fat reserve." To lose weight and reduce body fat, you need to tap into that reserve by reducing your calorie intake. Cutting calories doesn't mean sacrificing flavor. Enhancing the taste of lower-calorie meals is key to sticking with a healthier diet. Add herbs and spices to enhance the flavor. Choose sharp cheddar over mild cheddar because the sharper flavor will lead to eating less cheese. Try new foods—variety is a good thing. Maybe even try new cooking methods or recipes.

Cutting calories and losing weight boosts your overall health. It makes you feel more youthful, energetic, and even contributes to a longer, healthier life.

One effective strategy for cutting calories is to eat more nutrient-dense foods that are lower in calories. These include fruits, vegetables, whole grains, lean meats, poultry, egg whites, low-fat or fat-free dairy products, nuts, beans, and seeds. By prioritizing these foods, you can enjoy satisfying meals without overloading on calories, making it easier to achieve your health and weight-loss goals.

Adding Protein to Breakfast

Protein digests slowly, so it suppresses hunger hormones, and you feel full longer. Fifteen grams of protein at breakfast is a good start. Even minor amounts of protein reduce hunger pangs and cravings, which helps to shave off pounds! The benefit of eating a protein-rich breakfast is that you feel full longer and won't seek snacks before lunch. For years, we've heard that eating breakfast is essential for weight loss. To maximize this benefit, focus on incorporating protein into your first meal of the day.

A large egg contains about 6 grams of protein, so two eggs contain a good deal of protein to start your day. Other protein-rich possibilities are Greek yogurt, cottage cheese with fruit, a peanut butter and banana sandwich or toast, quinoa, or a tofu scramble. These choices not only deliver protein but also add variety and flavor to your morning routine, helping you stick to healthy eating habits.

Menopause and Possible Weight Gain

Let me put this as gently as possible. Going through perimenopause and menopause does not guarantee weight gain. They just don't. During this stage of life, declining estrogen levels can disrupt the balance between estrogen and progesterone, causing various symptoms such as irregular periods, mood swings, low libido, night sweats, hot flashes, vaginal dryness, and sometimes insomnia.

In terms of weight, the hormonal changes *may* make one more likely to gain weight around the waist, but hormonal changes *alone* don't cause weight gain. Lifestyle factors, such as diet and physical activity, as well as genetic predisposition, play a significant role.

Honestly, I wish menopause didn't even have a name—it's just another chapter in our lives, a natural progression of how our bodies evolve from the day we are born. Granted, there are changes that are annoying, even severe for some. Your body might feel out of control, and the fear of uncontrollable weight gain can loom large. This is a hot topic, creating a palpable fear among women of a certain age. However, it is a fact that not every woman gains weight as she ages.

It's true that change is happening, but it's not all bad. Sure, we're all going to experience symptoms. Maybe perimenopause starts with a 6-week-long period: bleeding, spotting, more spotting. The next step might be a uterine biopsy to rule out uterine cancer. Maybe there are night sweats, wet sheets, chills, feeling like you're in an oven. Of course, hot flashes happen, and they occasionally occur in our seventies! Yes, change is happening. While these experiences are real, they're not the entire story. In my professional opinion, it's about making lifestyle changes to help make the *change* tolerable.

One of my patients shared how she stopped feeling frustrated about her fatty middle and baggy clothes. Instead of going on another traditional diet—which rarely works—she made meaningful lifestyle changes, starting with small steps like reducing her sodium intake. Her success highlights the importance of focusing on lifestyle, not quick fixes. Here's how she approached her transformation:

- **Change Eating Habits**: She identified areas where she could improve her diet and made adjustments.

- **Choose Healthier Foods**: She swapped out less nutritious options for better choices.

- **Create an Exercise Routine**: She figured out a schedule that worked for her and stuck to it.

- **Practice Self-Compliments**: She celebrated her progress and body changes as the weight came off.

- **Set Goals and Celebrate Milestones**: Each achievement became a reason to celebrate, motivating her to keep going.

- **Maintain a Healthy Weight Range**: She focused on staying within a range that made her feel good.

- **Forgive Herself for Setbacks**: She didn't dwell on occasional backslides but got back on track without guilt.

Her journey shows that sustainable change comes from building habits that support long-term health and well-being, not short-term deprivation.

If we could strip away all the hype surrounding perimenopause and menopause and view it as another stage of life—a privilege for which we should be grateful—we might find it easier to embrace. Instead of battling against these natural changes, we can focus on adapting and committing to positive habits that support our well-being. By shifting the narrative from fear to empowerment, we can navigate this phase with grace and resilience, celebrating the strength that comes with each new chapter of life.

Lifestyle Changes for Sustainable Weight Management

Having a plan for weight loss or weight management saves time and money. Following a plan may also prevent you from eating unwanted calories. Most people plan meals on the weekend, so that they don't have to think about what to eat during the work week. My husband and I have been eating basically the same thing for almost two years: eloté and a salad. I know … that sounds crazy. What isn't crazy is that it requires little to no planning and I *love* that! I don't have to think about what to have for dinner every night. Sure, we add a piece of steak occasionally. Sometimes we eat out or get delivery, which is totally acceptable to do when you need a night off. An occasional dinner out won't wreck your entire weight loss plan. Because my husband must be on a soft food, liquid sort of diet, we have switched to eating soup. Once again, it's minimal meal planning. I make a big pot of pumpkin soup and voilà, we have meals for a few days! Same thing with potato soup, sweet potato soup, tomato soup … Planning reduces your scrounging around for food when you're hungry. It's a good idea to only have ingredients and foods in the house that are nutritious. Don't buy candy, chips, high-calorie foods, and high-fat snacks. Buy food like fruits and vegetables to snack on.

Keep a Gratitude Journal

Emotional eating, often triggered by stress, can lead to overeating and weight gain, with studies showing a link between mood disorders and obesity. Conditions such as depression and anxiety contribute to emotional and addictive eating, which can develop into an eating disorder. Emotional eaters choose high-calorie comfort foods over healthier options, leading to a higher Body Mass Index (BMI). However, weight reduction can improve overall well-being, enhance self-control, boost vitality, and reduce symptoms of depression and anxiety.

To break this unhealthy eating pattern, start a journal and write down the things you are grateful for. Studies show that people who express gratitude report healthier eating behavior over time. Journaling helps you cope with stress, the very thing that tempts you to reach for unhealthy foods.

Avoid Sugar or High Glycemic Foods

Sugar is a high-glycemic food, meaning it has a significant impact on blood sugar levels. The glycemic index measures how quickly foods raise blood sugar, with high-glycemic foods like refined white bread, white rice, crackers, doughnuts, cakes, and white potatoes, causing a rapid spike. However, this surge is quickly followed by a sharp drop, leading to hunger soon after consumption. Eating high-sugar, high-glycemic foods can leave you feeling hungry again almost immediately.

Eating too much sugar can also negatively affect your skin, leading to what's called "sugar sag." High sugar intake can also increase the free radicals in your body, damaging skin and promoting fine lines, wrinkles, and skin creping.

You can swap lower glycemic foods for the high glycemic ones: brown rice for white rice, whole grain bread for white bread, leafy greens for corn, and steel-cut oats for instant oatmeal.

Engage in Mindful Eating Practices

What is even meant by "mindful eating?" It means paying attention to the smell, texture, and taste of the food. Connect with your food. Look at it. Notice the colors and the smells before you even take the first bite. Think about where the food came from and how grateful you are to the growers and the Earth for the abundance of food you have in your kitchen.

People tend to eat without putting down their forks, so put down your fork between bites. This pause provides time for the body to recognize the "I am full" signal, reducing the possibility of overeating. Most of us ignore this signal and just keep eating because the food is in front of us, or we were taught to empty our plates. Early childhood messages can be very hard to ignore.

I know, I know … you've heard this all before. But remember, a plan only works if you stick to it, and it's even more effective when you have the right support and guidance.

Embracing a Healthy Weight for a Youthful Future

Maintaining a healthy weight is essential for staying vibrant, aging well, and preventing chronic conditions such as heart disease, high cholesterol, painful joints, and diabetes. Embracing gradual lifestyle changes, rather than overhauling everything at once, can make the journey more sustainable. Start with one small change, successfully implement it, and build on your progress. Be patient with yourself, celebrate every success—no matter how small—and stay committed to your well-being.

Incorporating principles from Chinese medicine can further support weight management and overall health. TCM addresses obesity-related conditions like asthma, sleep apnea, cardiovascular disease, hypertension, varicose veins, gallstones, kidney stones, chronic kidney disease, gout, back pain, sexual dysfunction, and acid reflux. TCM practitioners use a personalized approach based on an individual's unique imbalances, often related to qi stagnation, dampness, phlegm stagnation, and digestive issues involving the spleen and stomach.

A combination of acupuncture, herbal prescriptions, nutritional therapy, and lifestyle modifications is used to regulate metabolism, curb appetite, and reduce BMI. Studies show that acupuncture decreases inflammation, a common factor in obesity-related problems, while herbal remedies can help manage blood sugar, boost energy expenditure, and support gut health for improved digestion and weight maintenance. Additionally, practitioners may recommend stress-reducing activities such as tai chi or qigong to enhance sleep, ease anxiety and depression, and promote overall well-being.

By integrating these holistic approaches with mindful lifestyle changes, you can achieve and maintain a healthy weight, fostering long-term vitality and wellness.

BAD HABITS

CHAPTER 7

Make everything as simple as possible, but not simpler.

- Albert Einstein

THE WORLD HEALTH Organization emphasizes that preventing chronic diseases is rooted in healthy lifestyle choices and balanced diets, which can reduce the risk of these conditions by up to 80%. Traditional Chinese medicine also recognizes the importance of lifestyle and environmental factors, viewing health as a balance between inherited constitution and gained habits, such as diet and daily routines. Imbalances, including Yang deficiency, Yin deficiency, and Phlegm stasis, accelerate aging and lead to chronic health issues.

Unhealthy behaviors such as smoking, excessive alcohol consumption, late-night snacking, and a diet high in fried and fatty foods negatively impact both modern and traditional views of health. In Chinese medicine, these habits disrupt the body's natural energy balance, leading to weakened vitality and premature aging. Identifying and addressing these behaviors allows individuals to make informed choices that promote long-term wellness and disease prevention.

Whether viewed through the lens of modern medicine or traditional Chinese medicine, bad habits consistently impact health—each system may explain the effects differently, but the fundamental truth remains the same. Eliminating or reducing these harmful behaviors is essential for maintaining overall well-being and slowing the aging process.

Life's Worst Bad Habits

Smoking

We all know that smoking is linked to respiratory diseases, cardiovascular diseases, and various cancers, which all lead to premature death. The surgeon general published the first negative report on the consequences of smoking way back in 1964. The prevalence of smoking has gone down since then, but it's still the leading cause of preventable disease in the U.S.

Regarding external aging, smoking reduces blood flow to the skin, preventing oxygen and essential nutrients that nourish it. This damages collagen and elastin, leading to wrinkles, sagging skin, and an overall dull complexion. Eventually, smokers' lines form around the mouth and eyes, along with an uneven skin tone and hyperpigmentation (a.k.a. age spots).

Quitting smoking at any age is beneficial, but the earlier you stop, the greater the long-term health benefits. It's well established that non-smokers live significantly longer than those who smoke. If you're struggling to quit, consider these strategies to help you succeed:

- Set a quit date and prepare a quit plan.

- Seek support from friends, family, or support groups.

- If needed, use nicotine replacement therapies or prescribed medications.

- Identify and avoid smoking triggers.

Alcohol

Excessive alcohol consumption is strongly linked to liver disease, heart disease, addiction, pancreatic disorders, and premature death. The liver plays a crucial role in detoxifying the body, making it particularly vulnerable to damage from ethanol. One of the earliest and most common effects of heavy drinking is fatty liver disease, which results from excess fat accumulation in liver cells. While this condition is reversible with lifestyle changes, prolonged alcohol abuse can lead to cirrhosis—permanent scarring of the liver that can cause liver failure, requiring a transplant or leading to death. Reducing alcohol intake can significantly lower the risk of these life-threatening conditions and promote overall well-being.

Excessive alcohol consumption accelerates brain aging and significantly increases the risk of dementia. Over time, chronic drinking damages brain cells and reduces communication between neurons, leading to cognitive decline, memory loss, and difficulty with decision-making. While some short-term effects, like impaired coordination and slurred speech, may be temporary, long-term alcohol abuse can cause permanent brain damage. Studies show that heavy drinking contributes to brain shrinkage, particularly in middle-aged and older adults, increasing vulnerability to Alzheimer's disease and other forms of dementia. A shrinking brain is not only frightening but also impacts daily functioning, making it harder to maintain independence and mental clarity as you age. Reducing alcohol intake can help protect brain health, slow cognitive decline, and support long-term mental well-being.

Alcohol is dehydrating, leading to drier skin, wrinkles, puffy eyes, and broken capillaries, which make your skin look red and uneven. Dehydration reduces the skin's ability to retain moisture, causing it to lose elasticity and appear dull and saggy. Additionally, alcohol triggers inflammation, worsening conditions like rosacea and acne, while also impairing the body's ability to absorb essential nutrients such as vitamin A and collagen-building proteins. The long-term effects of alcohol on the skin contribute to premature aging, making fine lines and dark circles more pronounced. Cutting back on alcohol and staying hydrated can help maintain a more youthful, radiant complexion.

But how much alcohol is too much? The recommendation is 0.6 fluid ounces of pure alcohol, which is equal to one 12-ounce 5% alcohol beer, 8- or 9-ounce malt liquor, 5 ounces of wine, or a 1.5-ounce shot. Drink one per day for women or two for men. Heavy drinking means consuming more than three drinks per day for women or four for men. Alcohol can have both beneficial and harmful effects on health, depending on consumption levels. In moderation, such as small amounts of red wine, it has been linked to potential cardiovascular benefits due to antioxidants like resveratrol. However, excessive or frequent drinking can lead to severe health consequences already mentioned. The key to balancing alcohol's effects lies in mindful consumption and understanding its impact on overall well-being.

Red wine is a good option when choosing an alcoholic beverage, as it contains polyphenol antioxidants like resveratrol, which may offer benefits related to heart health, diabetes, some neurological conditions, and metabolic syndrome when consumed in moderation. Studies have shown that men who drank wine were 34% less likely to die early than those who drank beer or liquor. What is moderate? 1 to 2 glasses or less per day or a maximum of 7 per week for women and 14 per week for men.

QUICK NOTE

I couldn't find any studies suggesting that the benefits of moderate drinking outweigh the benefits of not drinking at all. So, don't view alcohol as a necessary health booster—there's no need to start drinking if you don't already.

If you're consuming too much alcohol, here are some things you can do to manage your alcohol consumption:

- Set limits on alcohol intake.

- Choose non-alcoholic beverages during social events.

- Seek support if you have trouble controlling alcohol consumption.

Lack of Activity

Skipping exercise is a harmful habit that leads to inactivity, which can negatively impact overall health and well-being. The health risks of physical inactivity include obesity, cardiovascular diseases, diabetes, and certain cancers. Lack of physical activity contributes to poor mental health and cognitive decline.

Lack of physical activity speeds up the signs of aging, affecting both appearance and overall health. Inactivity leads to a loss of muscle tone and strength, making everyday movements more difficult and increasing the risk of injury. Poor circulation can cause lifeless skin, as the body struggles to deliver essential nutrients and oxygen efficiently. Inactivity often contributes to increased fat deposition, particularly around the waist, which can further impact metabolism and overall well-being. Staying active helps maintain muscle strength, promotes healthy circulation, and supports a more youthful, vibrant body.

There is strong evidence that physical exercise positively alters brain plasticity, cognitive functioning, mood, and well-being. It is also a factor for reducing neurodegeneration. Physical exercise is an effective tool to reduce and prevent unhealthy behaviors like smoking, alcohol use, and gambling.

As we've already discussed, it's important to exercise in ways that keep you motivated. And it's important to remember that just going out for a brisk walk will help you maintain a healthy body weight and lose body fat that results in a healthier you.

Here are some other things you can do to stay fit:

- Find the activity you enjoy and are more likely to do regularly.

- Schedule regular exercise sessions into your daily routine.

- Set realistic fitness goals and track your progress.

Lack of Sleep

Getting enough sleep is a necessity because it improves brain performance, mood, and general health. On the other hand, lack of sleep increases the risk of high blood pressure, diabetes, depression, stroke, and obesity. Sleep deprivation may also weaken your immune system and lead to impaired cognitive function.

Insufficient sleep speeds up visible signs of aging, making your skin appear tired and less vibrant. Insufficient rest can lead to dark circles and puffiness under the eyes, a dull complexion, and an increase in fine lines. It also reduces skin elasticity, making it more prone to sagging and wrinkles, while slowing down the body's natural ability to heal wounds and repair damage. Prioritizing quality sleep is essential for maintaining a healthy, youthful glow.

Quality sleep isn't just about duration; it also includes sleep quality (uninterrupted and restful sleep) and maintaining a consistent sleep schedule. During sleep, the brain detoxifies itself, clearing out waste products that accumulate throughout the day, while the immune system undergoes essential repair and regeneration. Without sufficient rest, the body struggles to heal, fight infections, and maintain overall well-being as these crucial processes become disrupted. Prioritizing good sleep habits supports both physical and cognitive health, keeping you energized and resilient.

Screen time before bed disrupts sleep by interfering with the body's natural sleep cycle. Research shows that blue light from smartphones and tablets suppresses melatonin, the hormone that regulates sleep, making it harder to fall and stay asleep.

If you're having trouble sleeping, here are a few things you can do to improve the quality of your sleep:

- Establish a regular sleep schedule.

- Create a restful sleep environment (cool, dark, and quiet).

- Avoid screens and stimulants (caffeine, nicotine) before bedtime.

- Choose a mantra or breathing routine to relax.

Negative Self Talk

Sometimes, we are our own worst critics and struggle to find anything positive to say about ourselves. Our critical inner voice shouts out messages of doubt, fear, blame, and self-judgment. This has a negative impact on our mental and physical health. People who engage in frequent negative self-talk report feeling more stressed and anxious.

Negative self-talk contributes to chronic stress, increased cortisol levels, and poor mental health, all of which accelerate the aging process. Persistent self-criticism erodes self-esteem, making individuals more likely to engage in unhealthy behaviors, such as poor diet choices, lack of exercise, or substance use. This can lead to weight gain, increased inflammation, and higher risks of conditions like heart disease and diabetes—common factors in premature aging.

Stress from negative thinking impacts skin health by breaking down collagen and elastin, leading to wrinkles, dull skin, and premature sagging. Over time, this cycle of self-doubt and unhealthy habits not only affects physical appearance but also reduces overall longevity and well-being. Shifting to a more positive and self-compassionate mindset can help promote healthier lifestyle choices, reduce stress, and slow the aging process.

This may sound too simplistic, but while negative self-talk is associated with more stress, positive self-talk is a great predictor of success. Positive self-talk fosters resilience, improves problem-solving, and supports healthier lifestyle choices. Studies show that those who practice positive self-talk are more likely to achieve their goals and maintain overall well-being. Shifting to a growth-oriented mindset can boost confidence, reduce stress, and promote long-term success.

If you're feeling more negative than positive about your life, follow this advice:

- Catch your inner critic—it's easier to stop saying mean things to yourself when you notice it quickly.

- Treat yourself like you would a buddy. Would you say mean things to a friend?

- Practice mindfulness and self-awareness to catch negative thoughts.

- Use affirmations and positive statements.

Caffeine and Dehydration

Caffeine is a diuretic and leads to dehydration if consumed in excess, contributing to dry skin and the appearance of fine lines. Chronic dehydration affects the body's ability to flush out toxins, leading to a dull complexion, acne breakouts, or both. One of the most significant effects of caffeine on your skin is that it slows collagen production, which is essential for maintaining firmness and elasticity. Reduced collagen can lead to premature wrinkles and sagging, impacting overall skin health.

Speaking of aging, there is a surprising relationship between caffeine and age. It turns out that young people metabolize caffeine faster than adults over 65, so caffeine will stay in your body longer and prevent your ability to sleep if you drink caffeine too late in the day.

If you're drinking caffeinated drinks, be aware of these things:

- Notice if caffeine affects your sleep when you drink too much throughout the day or too late in the evening. If it does, try reducing your intake or adjusting the time of your last caffeinated drink.

- Replace caffeinated drinks with decaffeinated ones.

- Drink enough water throughout the day to stay properly hydrated.

Poor Makeup Application

While wearing makeup itself doesn't directly age your skin, be careful about the ingredients in the products you use. For example, added fragrances may cause irritation, especially if your skin is sensitive. Alcohol dries the skin and contributes to premature aging and the appearance of fine lines and wrinkles. Avoid products that contain parabens, propylene, PEGs, or other toxic ingredients.

The biggest makeup-related issues often stem from habits. Failing to remove makeup clogs pores, which can hinder collagen production and affect skin health. Less collagen leads to less elastic skin and then to wrinkles. Leaving it on overnight also allows the pollutants that have gotten on your skin during the day to sink deeper into your skin. Stretching your skin during application can cause irritation and loosen it. And using dirty brushes and applicators allows bacteria to accumulate.

Besides what has already been discussed, follow these best practices with your makeup:

- Don't use old makeup and replace it as needed.

- Apply sunscreen under makeup to protect your skin from premature aging and UV damage.

- Store makeup properly in a cool, dry place to prevent bacteria growth.

- Avoid sharing makeup to reduce the risk of infections, especially with eye and lip products.

Not Wearing Sunscreen

Wear sunscreen every day! Don't forget this step. Wearing sunscreen every day is crucial for protecting your skin from harmful ultraviolet (UV) radiation, which can cause short- and long-term damage. UV rays, even on cloudy or cool days, penetrate the skin, increasing the risk of premature aging, sunburn, and skin cancer. Daily sunscreen use creates a protective barrier that reduces these risks by blocking or absorbing UV radiation. Wearing sunscreen has so many positive results for your skin. Besides minimizing health risks, sunscreen helps maintain an even skin tone by preventing hyperpigmentation and sunspots. It also preserves the skin's natural elasticity by reducing collagen breakdown caused by UV exposure.

Here are the best practices when choosing and using sunscreen:

- Choose a broad-spectrum sunscreen with at least SPF 30 to ensure protection against both UVA (aging) and UVB (burning) rays.

- Regular application, even indoors, is vital because UV rays can penetrate windows. I remind people that your windshield does not act as a sunscreen.

- Incorporating sunscreen into your daily routine is a simple yet powerful habit for long-term skin health and youthful appearance.

Poor Oral Hygiene

Besides causing gum disease and tooth decay, poor oral health leads to inflammation, infection, and other serious illnesses such as heart disease, kidney disease, stroke, clogged arteries, problems with sexual health like erectile dysfunction and fertility challenges, osteoporosis, diabetes, and complications during pregnancy. As we've already covered, these conditions have a negative effect on overall aging and lifespan.

Poor oral hygiene may lead to acne, in that bad bacteria from your mouth migrates to the skin around your mouth, causing breakouts around your lips and on your chin. If those unhealthy bacteria from your mouth reach other areas of your face, there is a greater chance of skin inflammation and pimples. A good tip to remember is to wash your face after you brush your teeth.

Here are a few tips for good oral health:

- Brush your teeth in the morning and at night, and don't forget to floss daily.

- Reduce sugar intake to prevent tooth decay, cavities, and gum disease. This limits acid-producing bacteria that erode enamel and harm oral health.

- Use antiseptic mouthwash to kill bacteria, reduce plaque, and prevent bad breath and gum disease.

- Visit your dentist regularly for cleaning and annual exams.

Sitting More Than Standing

I saw an article that suggested sitting is the new smoking. Basically, sitting for long periods of time increases your risk of health problems such as diabetes, varicose veins, metabolic syndrome, heart disease, some cancers, and body aches like back problems. You could even experience mental-emotional issues like anxiety and depression.

When you think about it, humans were built to stand upright. This means that our systems work more effectively when we stand or move while in an upright position. Think about how people hospitalized and bedridden for extended periods of time develop difficulty with bowel movements. Extended time sitting or lying down weakens muscles, especially in our larger leg and butt muscles. It can also prevent our bones from maintaining strength. Deep vein thrombosis (DVT), a deep blood clot, starts from sitting for too long. Now airlines recommend moving around on long flights, even getting up from your seat and walking to avoid DVT. Lack of upright movement also causes aches and pains in the hips, lower back, neck, and shoulders.

A sedentary lifestyle affects your skin too. Blood pumps slower when you are less active. This means that your muscles and skin absorb fewer nutrients and oxygen, leading to premature aging of your skin.

People become less active as they age, but it's never too late to add physical activity to your day. It has *so* many health benefits!

Here are a few suggestions to mobilize your day:

- Walk 20 or 30 minutes each day.

- Take a lunch break outside and enjoy a walk in the fresh air. (Don't forget sunscreen.)

- If you have to drive to work, park a few blocks away and walk to the building.

- Use the stairs instead of the elevator or escalator.

- Take a class that includes movement, such as yoga or dance.

- Even standing instead of sitting helps, so stand while you read your emails or stand while you are on a conference call.

Breaking Bad Habits

Breaking bad habits takes awareness, effort, and patience, but it is entirely possible with the right approach. Whether it's smoking, unhealthy eating, or negative self-talk, repeated behaviors and triggers shape habits. By identifying what drives these habits and making intentional changes, you can gradually replace them with healthier alternatives. The process isn't about perfection—it's about progress. With the right strategies, support, and mindset, you can successfully break free from harmful patterns and build a healthier, more fulfilling lifestyle. Here are some essential steps to help you get started:

Identify the Bad Habit

- What specific habit do you want to change?
- How does this habit negatively impact your life?

Identify the Triggers

- When and where does this habit occur?
- What emotions or situations lead to this behavior?

Try to Reduce Those Triggers

- Can you avoid or minimize exposure to the trigger?
- What changes can you make to your environment to support success?

Replace the Bad Habit with a Healthier Activity

- What positive habit can take its place?
- How can you make this new habit easy and accessible?

Find Support

- Who can help keep you accountable?
- Would joining a group or working with a mentor/coach be helpful?

Visualize Success

- Can you picture yourself free from this habit?

- What benefits will you experience once you overcome it?

Be Patient with Yourself

- Are you allowing yourself time to make gradual progress?

- How will you handle setbacks without getting discouraged?

By following this checklist, you can take practical steps toward breaking bad habits and creating lasting, positive change.

Eliminating bad habits extends your lifespan, enhances your quality of life, and maintains your youthful appearance. By understanding the impact of bad habits, we take proactive steps to cultivate healthier habits. Embrace these changes with patience and persistence, and you will not only feel better but also look younger and more vibrant. Remember, aging is a natural process, and how gracefully we age is often within our control.

HAPPINESS

CHAPTER 8

> But if we are truly happy inside, then age brings
> with it a maturity, a depth, and a power that
> only magnifies our radiance.
>
> — David Deida

WHAT IS THIS thing called *happiness*, anyway? In the world of research, it's known as *positive affect* or a sense of *optimism*. Lyubomirsky defined it as, "An enduring state of mind consisting not only of feelings of joy, contentment, and other positive emotions, but also of a sense that one's life is meaningful and valued." *Psychology Today* stated, "It's a state of well-being that encompasses living a good life, one with a sense of meaning and deep contentment." The Greek Stoics said, "Happiness stemmed from being in control of one's own emotions." Harvard happiness expert Tal Ben-Shahar said, "Happiness lies at the intersection of pleasure and meaning." There is also a more generalized idea that happiness is a combination of how satisfied you are with your life, combined with how good you feel on a day-to-day basis.

No matter what the definition of happiness, feeling happy has a variety of positive effects on both your physical and mental health, and it may increase your longevity. In other words, happiness is a good thing. Interventions or therapies that promote happiness lead to better health and longevity outcomes. Happy people are healthier and live longer. This is because our bodies and minds are not separate, and mental health issues come with physical symptoms. Mind affects health.

Happy people live up to 18% longer than their less happy counterparts because happiness lowers our risk of heart disease and high blood pressure, enables more restful sleep, and allows us to maintain a healthy body weight along with regular exercise.

Negative attitudes and feelings of hopelessness create chronic stress but don't necessarily indicate classic signs of depression. Chronic stress upsets the body's hormone balance, reduces the brain chemicals required for happiness, and damages the immune system. It can also increase the risk of hypertension, heart attack, and stroke.

An unhappy person suffers from not feeling like herself and may feel helpless and hopeless, withdrawn from others, unable to take care of herself, or agitated. Unhappiness is called depression, and aches and pains are common with depression. Digestive problems, sleep disturbance, and appetite changes also accompany unhappiness. Any of these conditions can impact your health, immune system, and skin.

Why Are You Unhappy?

Your own well-being shouldn't be a mystery. The first thing to do is try to determine why you are unhappy. What is going on in your life? What is happening around you that makes you unhappy? Are you unsatisfied with your life choices? Do certain people make you unhappy? Once you figure out the root cause of your unhappiness, you're one step closer to addressing and overcoming it.

Research has confirmed that engaging in intentional practices will change the neural pathways in your brain. Scientists suggest that only 10% of happiness is because of external circumstances. The rest, the other 90% of our happiness, is based on our inner environment: thoughts and self-talk. *Wow!* This means mindfulness is highly trainable; we can retrain a negative thinking mind to be a positive thinking mind.

Things to Consider

These questions will help determine if your relationships and actions align with a happy life.

- **Who are the important people in your life and are you making time for them?** If you do not allocate time for significant individuals in your life, daily routines can become monotonous, and you may overlook what—or who— contributes to your well-being. Make sure you tell loved ones you love them. Set a scheduled time to call them once a week. I do this with one of my daughters—we obviously talk at other times too—but we expect to talk to each other every Tuesday morning.

- **Are you around too many negative people?** We feel the energy from the people around us and react to their behaviors. If the people around us are difficult to be around, we won't feel good; our energy drains. It's important to recognize and end toxic relationships. Surround yourself with people who are positive, supportive, and who feel good to be around.

- **What activities in life are important to you, and are you taking time to do them?** Prioritizing activities that bring you joy, fulfillment, and relaxation is essential for maintaining happiness and well-being. Whether it's spending time with loved ones, pursuing creative hobbies, exercising, or simply enjoying nature, making space for these moments can significantly improve your mood and reduce stress. Consider when you feel most content—what activities make you lose track of time because they are engaging? Identifying these passions and making them a priority can have a powerful impact on your well-being. If you find yourself constantly caught up in responsibilities, try scheduling time for the things that matter most to you. Whether it's something that excites you, helps you focus, or simply brings you peace, dedicating time to what you love will enhance your daily life and overall happiness. Small, intentional changes can lead to a more balanced and satisfying life.

- **Are you feeling like a failure?** Ask if you are trying to live up to *your* idea of success or someone else's. Expectations matter in relationships, including our relationship with ourselves. Define what success means to you personally and what expectations you have of yourself. Work at meeting your own standards rather than those of others or some vague social expectations.

- **Are you taking care of your body?** Physical health is linked to mental health. Minor changes in how you take care of your body may have a big impact on your happiness. Prioritize getting enough high-quality sleep in your daily routine. Take a walk and absorb some sunshine. Exercise regularly. Eat a healthy balanced diet, snacking wisely. Take deep breaths. Drink enough water to stay hydrated …

- **Do you say "yes" too often because you feel obligated or pressured?** Overcommitting to others can leave you feeling drained and overwhelmed. Start by saying "no" to small requests—it will get easier over time. If you don't have the time or availability, try responding with, "I'm busy at that time, so I can't help out," or simply, "I'm sorry, I can't help this time." Setting boundaries allows you to balance your commitments while making space for your own self-care and well-being.

How to Improve Happiness

While the definition of happiness varies across cultures and individuals, happiness is commonly linked to positive relationships, personal achievements, and a sense of purpose. Happiness is not the absence of negative emotions; it's a proactive pursuit of mental, emotional, and physical well-being. It encompasses both fleeting pleasures, such as savoring a good meal, and lasting fulfillment, like building meaningful connections or pursuing a passion. Research shows that happiness is shaped by genetics, life circumstances, and personal choices. To improve your happiness, consider the following strategies:

Get Up and Move

Physical activity reduces emotional stuckness by reducing levels of stress hormones like cortisol and by releasing endorphins, our "happy brain" chemicals. Exercise also helps us feel stronger, improves self-image, and renews vigor in life. In Chinese medicine, we know that exercise moves overall energy, keeping emotional energy moving rather than allowing it to get stuck and lead to anxiety or depression. Plus, heavier breathing during exercise helps our body better utilize oxygen. Any exercise works: walking, running, weight training, swimming …

As I've mentioned, find something you *enjoy* doing. For me it's running, even though I once hated the activity. When I played soccer, I'd run in between matches to stay fit. When the pandemic halted soccer, I dinked around with a combination of running and walking to stay fit—I called them 'run walks.' I even bought appropriate shoes and took running lessons. Now I am literally in love with running! So, things change. Find what's perfect for you!

Give to a Charity

Donating to charity or giving gifts to others is called "prosocial spending." Whatever you do to benefit others increases the giver's happiness level. Choosing and giving a gift to someone rather than buying something for yourself also results in a euphoric feeling. Human beings experience emotional rewards from rewarding others. Find a cause that you care about and contribute to it with your time, money, or resources.

Look at Life with Gratitude

Research says that gratitude can significantly improve your health and happiness. For one thing, being grateful shifts your focus from what you think is lacking in your life to what is abundant in your life. Start a gratitude practice or perspective.

Keeping a gratitude journal or sharing good things about your day is simple. Live by the adage of counting your blessings! Be grateful for a beautiful day in the park, watching kids play. Appreciate a random act of kindness, such as someone letting you cut the line at the grocery store. List literally anything you feel grateful for.

Gather a clear, empty jar and some colorful pieces of colored paper and make a gratitude jar. When something good happens, write it down and put it in the jar. When you walk by the jar, you'll see a pretty flash of colors, reminding you about the good things that happen. You'll have lots to be grateful for.

Be Calm and Collected

Start practicing meditation. Usually, I don't use the word "meditation" with my patients when we talk about calming down, reducing stress, and getting healthier. I simply tell them, "Meditation equals focus—that's it." It's not mumbo jumbo, extra spiritual, or difficult to perfect. Meditation is merely focus. It rewires your brain, creating a calmer, friendlier mind. The ability of our brains to meditate is called neuroplasticity, and it includes two processes: 1) neurogenesis, which is the growth of new neurons and 2) synaptogenesis, which is the creation of connections between neurons.

Focus or meditate in a way that suits you. Chanting is one of my favorite ways to focus. When I focus on words during a chant, I'm not thinking about stressful situations. And chanting provides a way to exercise our lungs and better utilize oxygen. But for you, maybe it's mindfulness or breathing exercises.

View Happy Photos

Happiness is so subjective and how to feel it varies from person to person. For example, if you have a smart phone, bringing up the photo app is a reminder of your happy moments in seconds. My husband is an expert at reliving happy memories, and me, not so much. Some pictures from the past—even ones of very, very happy times—make me cry. It's because I feel sorry that those times are over. So, I made a change. I only add pictures that make me smile to device backgrounds and slideshows. For other happy times photos, I follow the tried-and-true three-step happy memory psychological process: enjoying the planning, the doing, and the memories! As I said, I'm still not perfect at the third, enjoying the memories, but I'm working on it.

Smile

Did you know that the physical act of smiling can actually make you feel happier? Research shows that engaging the facial muscles used to smile—even by holding a pencil between your teeth—triggers the brain to release feel-good chemicals, signaling happiness. To boost your mood, surround yourself with things that bring joy, like a playlist of uplifting music, a collection of funny videos, or a gratitude journal filled with positive memories. You can also create a "happiness corner" with favorite photos, keepsakes, or inspiring quotes. When you engage with these joyful reminders, your brain reinforces feelings of happiness, helping to lift your spirits even on tough days.

Express Emotions

I tell my patients that emotions are better expressed than held in. When we hold our emotions in, we stagnate, and they build until they burst out, sometimes in a bad way. There's no need to become raging maniacs. What I mean is that emotions need to be acknowledged and expressed rather than suppressed. If you feel like crying, take a few minutes to cry. If you feel frustrated or angry, express it constructively. You can express it in private; you don't have to hold a grudge. Holding our emotions in is what results in physical symptoms. The Masters said, "Emotions cause all physical disease." I heard this saying during my first week in Chinese medicine school and didn't give it much credence. But as the years of schooling progressed, I saw what they meant: holding in emotions creates the stagnation of energy that will eventually turn into physical symptoms.

Connect with People

Building and maintaining strong social relationships is crucial for happiness. An eighty-year study by a Harvard research group concluded that happiness is all about relationships. One of the study's directors, Dr. Robert Waldinger, said, "Relationships and how happy we are in those relationships have a powerful effect on our health." He also felt that loneliness was as dangerous to our health as smoking or alcoholism.

The study revealed that close relationships keep people happy throughout their lives, more so than money or fame. Close, satisfying relationships delay mental and physical decline. They are also better predictors of one having a long, happy life than social class, IQ, or even genetic makeup.

Researchers identified several key factors that contribute to healthy aging, including regular physical activity, not smoking, minimal alcohol intake, maintaining a healthy weight, stable marriage, effective coping mechanisms, and education. However, above all, strong relationships matter most—relationships, relationships, relationships. Strong, supportive connections with others play the biggest role in long-term well-being and longevity.

Learn Something New

Studies show that mental decline with age is not a given. The brain is like a muscle: if you don't exercise regularly, its ability to function will decline. And mental exercise isn't the only exercise that has anti-aging effects on your brain. Staying physically active does too!

Just how muscles increase in size with exercise, according to the *National Institute on Aging*, so does the part of your brain that is important for memory and learning. Research is being conducted on many activities to see how staying active and engaged changes the brain. Quilting, digital photography, dancing, theater, regular internet calls with family or friends, doing volunteer work, and walking with a group have all shown promise to lower the risk of cognitive decline with age. We are better able to do many things with overall positive brain health. We think, learn, and remember more, and we are better able to maintain a good sense of balance and ability to control our body's movements. A healthy brain efficiently processes emotions, and our senses are stronger.

One of the significant advantages of learning later in life is the freedom to choose courses that genuinely interest you, rather than those dictated by a school curriculum. Thanks to technology, you can now take courses from the comfort of your home at your own pace or opt for hybrid classes that combine online and in-person learning. With greater discipline and improved time management skills compared to your teenage years, you're likely to be more successful in your studies. Set a goal to learn a new skill every year—it's a great way to stay engaged, challenged, and continuously grow.

Happiness = Longevity

Happiness is a crucial component of overall well-being and longevity. By understanding the factors that contribute to unhappiness and actively working to incorporate habits that promote joy, individuals can significantly improve their quality of life. Remember that happiness is a journey, not a destination. It's about making daily choices that align with your values and bring you closer to a state of contentment and fulfillment.

With Traditional Chinese Medicine (TCM), when someone comes to my office complaining of depression, my first step is to determine the root cause of their unhappiness. Through conversation, I explore whether they are experiencing grief from a recent loss, lingering sadness from childhood, or if they need to make significant life changes. Identifying the underlying issue is crucial in guiding the healing process.

For those dealing with grief, there is a natural process of mourning that must be honored. If unresolved childhood sadness resurfaces, I help them implement techniques to improve happiness, as mentioned earlier. In cases where life changes are necessary, we work together to identify steps that bring balance and fulfillment.

As a practitioner, my primary goal is to restore the person's energy flow to the heart and spirit, making it vibrant and free once again. Acupuncture and herbal medicine nurture the spirit, offering support as individuals navigate life's challenges. I also use specialized acupuncture treatments to help release old trauma patterns when someone feels stuck in past pain.

It's truly rewarding to witness people reconnect with their essence of happiness. If you are seeking a way to rediscover joy and emotional balance, consider exploring Chinese medicine—it may offer the support and healing you need.

OPTIONS

CHAPTER 9

My face carries all my memories. Why would I
erase them?

- Diane Von Furstenberg

I'M ALWAYS FASCINATED by how far people will go to chase youth and
beauty. In this chapter, we'll explore various cosmetic procedures available today, along with their potential risks and side
effects. When you see the complications of certain treatments,
the idea of getting a minor bruise from something like Cosmetic
Acupuncture will seem mild by comparison.

Honestly, the best procedure for you depends on your specific
skin care goals. Are you looking to reduce age spots or even out
your complexion? Maybe you want to enhance your skin's ability
to retain moisture. Perhaps your focus is on healing your skin to
prevent future acne breakouts, or you're searching for an effective
way to minimize wrinkles and achieve a natural lift.

For lifting, wrinkle reduction, and treating acne scars, my
favorite tool is the acupuncture needle. With my knowledge of
the dermis's depth, I can precisely place the needle where it will
be most effective. Acupuncture is unique because it works with

your body's natural healing processes to stimulate collagen and elastin production, helping you achieve the results you want in a natural and sustainable way.

In the following sections, we'll explore a variety of skin care treatments, from non-invasive options to more intensive procedures, so you can make an informed decision about what works best for you.

Filler Injections

As you know, these days we have a slew of injectable choices that promise to plump up skin, reduce lines between the eyebrows, fill in the area under the eyes, puff up lips, flatten nasolabial grooves, and more. The very first injectable filler approved by the FDA was called Zyderm collagen, and it was made from cowhides. Since collagen injections have traditionally been made from cow or pig parts, they require allergy testing before the injections are administered. But now we have injections of human collagen that may not require allergy testing. Results from the injections are temporary, and side effects are usually minimal but include swelling, redness, irritation, and changes in skin color.

The most natural injections are microlipo injections, autologous fat injections, or autologous fat transfer, which means they use your own fat. Sometimes, people joke about these procedures by saying, "It looks like your butt is on your face." Essentially, fat is taken from an area with excess and transferred to the face. The process begins with liposuction under local anesthesia to harvest fat cells. The fat is first processed to remove excess fluids and thoroughly cleaned before being injected into its new location. Yes, that means fat from the butt or belly gets transferred to the face! Don't worry, you don't have to have liposuction before each injection. They typically remove excess fat and freeze it for future use.

This injection is considered safe because it uses the patient's own fat, eliminating the risk of allergic reactions and the need for allergy testing. It is also known for delivering longer-lasting results compared to other fillers. Common side effects include swelling, redness, and bruising at the injection sites, but these usually fade within a few days.

Restylane and Juvederm are fillers made of hyaluronic acid, a substance our body naturally produces to maintain skin volume and fullness. Synthetic hyaluronic acid was discovered in the 1930s, and NASHA (Non-Animal-Stabilized Hyaluronic Acid) is a non-animal-derived form used in cosmetic treatments to reduce signs of aging. There are those who think that Restylane is the synthetic answer to our natural decline because injections of it add fullness to areas and/or reduce the prominence of wrinkles. Results may last six months or longer, which is a decent time for fillers. One reason for this may be because hyaluronic acid attracts and binds to water, helping the fullness last longer. Side effects may include bruising, redness, pain, itching, tenderness, swelling, infection, allergic reactions, bumps, necrosis, and acne.

Botulism Toxin Injections

The results from Botulism toxin injections, more commonly known as Botox®, are temporary, which means making trips to a physician, dermatologist, or other specialist for additional injections once the effects wear off. The injections are not without risk, yet they remain an extremely popular cosmetic treatment. I've heard Botox® referred to as a "muscle poison" because it works by blocking nerve impulses to the muscles responsible for frowning, squinting, and pursing the lips. In theory, if you can't make facial expressions, you won't form wrinkles. Unfortunately, long-term use of Botox® may cause muscles to become so relaxed that they lose their ability to create certain facial expressions. This should be a concern, along with one of the immediate side effects, frequent headaches.

The paralyzing effects of the Botox® sometimes migrate to an area close to the injection site, creating unwanted results. I had a patient call me crying because she couldn't make facial expressions after receiving Botox® injections. Of course. Inability to make facial expressions is one of the side effects listed in the warnings. I guess she didn't read the potential effects before her injections. While she was upset, she refused an acupuncture treatment because she didn't want to stop the effects of the Botox®. Wait, I thought she wanted to make facial expressions, so I told her to wait 3 to 6 months for the effects to wear off.

I once had a patient who received Botox® injections for crow's feet on one side of her face, but the paralyzing effect unintentionally spread to her eyelid, preventing her from closing her eye voluntarily. As a result, she had to tape her eyelid shut at night just to sleep. She came to me, hoping to reverse the effects of the Botox®. Fortunately, through Cosmetic Acupuncture, I was able to stimulate blood flow and oxygen circulation throughout her face, and soon, she regained the ability to close her eyelid naturally.

When considering treatments like Botox®, it's important to weigh the benefits against the potential risks. While these procedures can provide a smoother, more youthful appearance, they also come with side effects that may impact facial movement and expression. Understanding how these treatments work and exploring alternative options, such as Cosmetic Acupuncture, can help you make an informed decision about what's best for your long-term well-being. Ultimately, maintaining healthy skin through good skin care, hydration, and non-invasive treatments can often provide natural, lasting results without the risks associated with injectables.

Laser Treatments

Laser treatments, also known as laser peel and laser vaporization, use light energy to generate heat. The laser machine emits short, concentrated pulsating beams of light into the skin, precisely removing it layer by layer. These treatments vaporize the epidermis (the outer layers of skin), sloughing off dead skin and revealing a smooth, new layer. The goal is to target the dermis to eliminate age spots and other discolorations. After all, the dermis is where real changes occur, making it the key to achieving lasting and dramatic anti-aging results.

Older ablative laser models require a local anesthetic, sometimes combined with an IV-administered sedative (conscious sedation), to minimize discomfort. Additionally, patients need an ointment to prevent scab formation and a sterile dressing on the treated areas for 24 hours. These treatments take anywhere from 10 to 21 days to heal. The skin looks badly sunburned for a couple of days before peeling for up to 10 days.

There are several types of laser treatments available, each designed to address specific skin concerns with varying levels of intensity and downtime. Understanding these different treatment options can help determine the best approach for achieving long-term skin rejuvenation.

Ablative Lasers

While the old-fashioned ablative lasers caused epidermal burning, the more recent, less invasive non-ablative lasers distribute heat into the dermis without causing outward burning, so the epidermis remains intact. The thermal energy penetrates the dermis to stimulate collagen without making the outer layers of skin look burned. The face is still red for a few days after the procedure and needs special care, but the overall potential for scarring is much lower with the newer lasers.

Fraxel Lasers

Fraxel lasers target specific areas of the skin in a controlled pattern, creating microscopic injuries while leaving surrounding tissue intact to promote faster healing and collagen production. Therein the name "Fraxel" for "fractional" treatment. This sort of procedure leaves areas of the skin untouched, resulting in a more natural look and the face doesn't look so completely red or burned afterward. These treatments target damaged tissue in the dermis and leave the outer layers of skin (the epidermis) relatively unaffected. Treating the dermis leads to deeper and longer lasting healing. The treatment requires local anesthesia and occasionally a pain management plan. The treatment plan is generally 3 to 5 treatments that are spaced about 4 weeks apart. Swelling and redness may occur but fades within a few days. Infection and scarring are very rare.

Titan Lasers

Titan laser treatments improve collagen production and architecture. Results usually develop over time, so there is a waiting period of up to six months to see the maximum results. The procedure treats sagging skin anywhere on the body because it doesn't injure fat in the skin like some lasers do. The treatment may feel hot, and there may be some mild pain, discomfort, redness, and swelling, but there is no real downtime. Multiple treatments are necessary, and the results last about two years.

Skin Tyte

Another non-invasive light energy treatment is Skin Tyte. This system delivers light energy (heat) treatment with better skin cooling technology. It simultaneously heats the dermis (the deeper layers of your skin) while cooling the outer layers (epidermis). The treatment is applied on the face, neck, hands, chest, and arms to freshen the look of skin. They often claim there's no downtime and that the procedure is painless, though numbing creams are available in case of discomfort. Some mild swelling may occur for a day or two, along with occasional bruising or blistering, but these side effects typically resolve quickly. Some people get hyperpigmentation that requires additional treatment. The results may last for up to six months. Multiple treatments are necessary, and follow-up treatments are recommended. If that's not enough *drama*, here's a list of potential side effects:

- milia (small white bumps)
- hyperpigmentation (dark spots)
- hypopigmentation (white or light spots)
- cold sores (take antiviral medication before laser treatment)
- bacterial infections
- swelling, scarring

The dermatologist or surgeon may also recommend sleeping on an extra pillow to reduce the potential for swelling. And stop smoking to minimize the risk of complications and support the healing process.

Intense Pulsed Light Treatment

IPL (Intense Pulsed Light) treatment is also known as light laser, photo laser, or photo facial. If laser resurfacing sounds like too much for you, that's still what you are receiving. The newer lasers are a modification of the original laser resurfacing. The treatments specifically target damaged skin and broken capillaries in the dermis. Intense light energy penetrates the skin, where it is absorbed by dilated blood vessels, effectively reducing their appearance. The heat of the laser causes damage in the dermis that stimulates collagen synthesis as the body begins the healing process. The healing period for this treatment is much faster than for traditional laser resurfacing, but several treatments are usually required. Four to six treatments spaced about four weeks apart are recommended. Most people feel a little heat and stinging, and their skin appears a little red, but recipients typically continue a normal day after treatment. They say that side effects are rare but may include blistering and slight bleeding, possible permanent hypopigmentation or hyperpigmentation, and, very rarely, scarring. By the way, scars are permanent. Some people need a treatment every three weeks for some months.

A Case to Consider Before Undergoing a Laser Treatment

I had a patient who underwent laser treatments on her neck to reduce redness. She had a distinct "necklace" pattern where the skin under her chin, untouched by the sun, remained lighter than the rest. The laser practitioner recommended three sessions, explaining that multiple treatments were needed for optimal results.

The first two treatments went smoothly, but during the third session, she told the practitioner that she felt a burning or sparking sensation—unlike her previous experiences. The practitioner assured her there was nothing to worry about since the same settings were being used as before. However, it was later discovered that the laser had been repaired between her second and third treatments, and when it was returned, it was working more powerfully than before.

Immediately after the session, her neck turned bright red—essentially burned—and she broke out in hives. The clinic provided an ice pack for the ride home and later advised her to apply Cortisone cream when the itching and hives persisted. Soon after, the area became scabby, leaving her anxious about potential scarring. Fortunately, once the scabs healed, no scars remained. However, for nearly a year, she continued to break out in hives whenever she sweated.

This experience serves as an important reminder—always ask your laser professional about potential risks and inquire about any equipment changes that might affect your treatment.

Microdermabrasion

Dermabrasion is a true surgical procedure and could have significant side effects, including scarring. It was once done under general anesthesia while a surgeon sanded down the skin. Because of the dangers of anesthesia, there is now microdermabrasion. The procedure still sands off the skin, but it penetrates much less deeply than dermabrasion.

Many aestheticians offer this procedure, and it's typically sold in packages containing several treatments. Again, be certain to find a qualified aesthetician if you are interested in microderm-abrasion because side effects like hyper- or hypopigmentation may occur. Depending upon the depth of the treatment, your skin may feel sensitive or achy afterward. To actually see anti-aging results, you may need up to a dozen or so treatments over a weekly, bi-monthly, or monthly time period.

After a few days of swelling, redness, and a stinging sensation, my patient's skin tone appeared more even, and her complexion looked noticeably rejuvenated. However, the effects were temporary, and regular follow-up treatments were needed to maintain the results.

Chemical Peels

Chemical peels burn off the outer layers of skin to reveal the younger, smoother skin below. Back in the early 1900s, the first recorded chemical peel included phenol: a peeling agent derived from coal tar. It's basically a controlled exfoliation or controlled burn.

I am what aestheticians call a "chemical peel weenie." I don't like to feel even a slight burning sensation on my skin. An aesthetician says, 'tingly.' I say, "burny." Despite that, I trust my aesthetician to take me on a safe, comfortable exfoliation journey using very, very gentle chemical peels—as gentle as possible for a burning chemical.

A glycolic acid peel is considerably superficial, so it only makes a slight difference in reducing wrinkles. Deeper peels use ingredients like salicylic or trichloroacetic acid. After receiving a chemical peel, it is a big no-no to go out in the sun because sun exposure causes hyperpigmentation. In fact, you may need to hide out for a few days because your face looks burned. Your face may feel sore, like sunburn, and peel for a few days. But the treatment results in much smoother skin, and some fine lines may even disappear.

Again, be certain to choose a skilled, ethical aesthetician, and make sure you fully understand the treatment you are receiving. I had a patient who received what she called a "green peel" during her course of Cosmetic Acupuncture treatments. She came in for her third treatment with a red, peeling, sore face. Naturally, I couldn't do Cosmetic Acupuncture that day; I don't work on burned or raw skin because there could be an infection. And the acupuncture would be painful because her skin was already hurting. She was basically shocked by her soreness and peeling because of the name "green" and the label "organic." I explained to her that it's still a peel; it's still a burn.

Thermage

Some people consider Thermage to be the only non-invasive procedure that produces tighter skin. Thermage uses radio waves to heat the dermis and underlying tissue, causing collagen to tighten and stimulate new collagen production. The heat thickens collagen, leading to smoother, tighter-looking skin. When the body senses damage, it starts the wound-healing process, creating new collagen in the affected areas. Typically, you only need one treatment for results, but visible results take four to six months. It's the dermis that is targeted and affected, so the outer skin remains intact. I've heard that it hurts, but the literature I've read states that the only sensations are suction and maybe some heat. This means there is virtually no downtime except for some swelling.

I've only known one person who had Thermage, and she described the procedure as slightly painful with some swelling. She chose not to follow up with additional treatments and felt the results were minimal.

Surgery

There is no shortage of anti-aging surgical procedures, including facelifts (rhytidectomy), upper and lower eyelid lifts (blepharoplasty), brow lifts, chin and cheek implants, Gore-Tex implants, and even tendon grafts for lip enhancement—the list goes on. The thing about surgery is that it's serious business. While exact statistics on botched cosmetic surgeries may be hard to find, high-profile cases are often featured on talk shows discussing surgical mishaps or can easily be found through a quick internet search. And even though serious complications are infrequent, negative side effects do occur with almost any procedure. Heck, even with acupuncture, you might get a bruise. But the negative side effects of a surgery gone bad are more noticeable, more dangerous, and potentially longer lasting than a bruise. Ugly scarring or numbness are the *least* of your worries, and death is the *worst* of your worries when considering surgery.

I treated a woman whose jaw was numb for two years after her facelift. Cosmetic Acupuncture restored the feeling. Pretty cool. Remember that surgical facelift results only last from six to eight years because the clock is still ticking, and gravity continues to pull the skin downward. Understandably, this woman never had another surgery; one was enough for her.

Microneedling

The purpose of microneedling is to generate new collagen and skin tissue for a smoother and more toned skin. According to research, skin treated with four microneedling sessions spaced one month apart produced up to a 400% increase in collagen and elastin six months after completing treatment.

Microneedling uses a specialized device with fine, short needles that penetrate the skin, stimulating collagen production when applied at a depth that reaches the dermis. It reduces wrinkles and fine lines, stimulates hair regrowth, decreases acne scarring, improves or prevents sagging, and smooths the skin's overall tone and appearance.

The protocol is a series of three treatments several weeks apart. You will also see long-term results when you receive a few treatments a year for maintenance.

My patients like to schedule their microneedling on Fridays because their skin is red and swollen after a treatment. This allows their skin to calm down before returning to work on Monday. It's an excellent treatment for overall skin rejuvenation, but since it doesn't penetrate very deeply, it's not typically effective for erasing deep lines or wrinkles. However, it can help improve skin texture and reduce the appearance of minor acne scars.

Radiofrequency (RF) Skin Tightening

RF skin tightening uses an electromagnetic device to heat the skin and stimulate collagen production, resulting in firmer, tighter skin. It is mainly used to treat sagging skin. This non-invasive treatment can be applied to both the face and body, offering minimal downtime and gradual, natural-looking results. However, the effects are temporary, typically lasting one to two years. Potential side effects include pain, swelling, and redness.

A patient of mine received RF skin tightening on her abdomen post-pregnancy. She reported noticeable skin tightening over a few months, with no significant side effects.

Ultherapy

Ultherapy uses focused ultrasound energy to lift and tighten the skin on the face, neck, and décolletage. It targets deeper layers of the skin, promoting collagen regeneration with no downtime. Results can take several months to fully develop.

One of my patients underwent Ultherapy for sagging skin on her neck and noticed a gradual lifting effect over six months, with minimal discomfort during the procedure.

Cryolipolysis (CoolSculpting)

CoolSculpting is a non-invasive fat reduction treatment that uses controlled cooling to freeze and eliminate fat cells. It is commonly used on areas like the abdomen, thighs, and flanks. The body naturally processes and eliminates the dead fat cells over time.

A patient opted for CoolSculpting on her love handles. She experienced mild discomfort during the procedure and slight bruising afterward, but she was pleased with the reduction in fat after a few months.

Chinese Medicine Options for Anti-Aging

Chinese medicine is primarily a preventive medicine. That is, you start treatments before you have symptoms, while you are young, to keep your immune system strong, digestion working well, sleeping patterns normal, etc. I like to remind people that Chinese medicine is the true anti-aging medicine because, when you are healthy and treat your skin naturally, you will age well. Here are some of the Chinese medicine treatments for anti-aging.

Acupuncture for Health

As I've mentioned, staying strong and healthy is key to aging gracefully. One effective way to achieve this is by receiving regular acupuncture treatments. Acupuncture, a key component of traditional Chinese medicine, has been practiced for thousands of years to promote overall health and well-being. It restores balance, alleviates blockages, and supports the body's natural healing mechanisms.

One significant way acupuncture improves general health is by reducing stress and promoting relaxation. It encourages the release of endorphins, the body's natural painkillers, and serotonin, a hormone that regulates mood. This helps reduce anxiety, improve sleep quality, and enhance mental clarity.

Acupuncture is also known to boost immune function. By stimulating specific acupoints, it enhances the production of white blood cells and strengthens the body's ability to fight off infections. Additionally, it helps regulate the autonomic nervous system, balancing the "fight or flight" response with the "rest and digest" state, fostering overall physiological harmony.

Beyond immune support, acupuncture improves circulation, reduces inflammation, and addresses chronic pain—factors critical to maintaining good health. Regular sessions may also help prevent illness by supporting organ function and maintaining homeostasis, ensuring a healthier, more balanced lifestyle.

Cosmetic Acupuncture

I practice and teach a specific form of cosmetic acupuncture called Mei Zen, which means "beautiful person" because I treat your whole body. The goal is to keep your body healthy and work on your facial and/or neck skin at the same time. The needles stimulate fibroblasts of collagen and elastin to improve the skin and reduce wrinkling.

In addition to its aesthetic benefits, Mei Zen Cosmetic Acupuncture also enhances overall well-being by promoting circulation, balancing hormones, and reducing stress. By improving blood flow and oxygenation to the skin, this technique supports a natural, radiant complexion without the need for invasive procedures. Many patients also report experiencing improved sleep, better digestion, and a greater sense of relaxation because of the holistic approach. Unlike treatments that only focus on external appearance, Mei Zen works from the inside out, ensuring long-term results that reflect both inner and outer vitality.

Facial Gua Sha

Facial Gua Sha is a form of Chinese medical massage that offers numerous benefits to your skin. The massage is done with various Gua Sha tools made from natural stones like jade and rose quartz. By using this smooth-edged tool to gently massage the face, Gua Sha promotes blood circulation, enhancing your skin's natural glow. It helps to relieve tension in facial muscles, reducing puffiness and the appearance of fine lines. Regular practice can improve lymphatic drainage, eliminate toxins, and promote a firmer, more sculpted complexion. Gua Sha also boosts product absorption, maximizing the effectiveness of serums and oils. Beyond the physical benefits, it provides a soothing, meditative experience, reducing stress and supporting overall well-being. To incorporate Gua Sha into your skin care routine, start with a clean face and apply a facial oil or serum to allow the tool to glide smoothly over the skin. Some key exercises include:

- **Neck Release**: Glide the tool from the base of your neck up toward your jawline to encourage lymphatic drainage.

- **Jawline Sculpting**: Use the edge of the tool to gently scrape along the jawline, moving outward from the chin to the ear. This helps to reduce tension and define the jawline.

- **Cheek Lifting**: Starting from the sides of your nose, sweep the tool along your cheekbones toward your temples to promote a lifted appearance.

- **Under-Eye Depuffing**: Using the curved edge, lightly glide from the inner corner of your eye toward the temples to reduce puffiness and improve circulation.

- **Forehead Smoothing**: Move the tool in upward strokes from your eyebrows to the hairline to help release tension and soften fine lines.

For best results, practice Gua Sha a few times a week or daily, depending on your skin's needs. Consistency will help you achieve a more sculpted, radiant, and rejuvenated appearance.

Herbal Masks

Chinese herbal masks have long been used to nourish and rejuvenate the skin, offering a natural approach to skin care that addresses a variety of concerns. Certain Chinese herbs, like Huang Qi (astragalus), improve skin elasticity and promote a healthy glow by boosting circulation and collagen production. Seaweed (hai dai) is another commonly used ingredient, rich in minerals and antioxidants that help detoxify the skin, reduce redness, and improve hydration.

Herbs are carefully selected based on individual skin needs, whether for reducing inflammation and acne breakouts, providing deep hydration, or offering anti-aging benefits. For example, bai zhi (angelica root) helps brighten the complexion and fade dark spots, while gou qi zi (goji berry) is packed with vitamins that enhance skin repair and fight oxidative stress. Yu zhu (Solomon's Seal) is known for its deeply moisturizing properties, making it ideal for dry or aging skin.

To use herbal masks effectively, the powdered herbs are often mixed with natural bases like honey, yogurt, rice water, or green tea to create a smooth paste that is applied to the skin. Some masks may also include pearl powder for skin brightening or licorice root for its soothing and anti-inflammatory effects.

When applied regularly, herbal masks can help restore balance to the skin, providing long-term benefits without the harsh chemicals found in many commercial skin care products. Whether aiming to reduce wrinkles, clear up acne, or enhance hydration, these herbal treatments offer a time-tested solution for achieving naturally radiant skin.

While I highlighted the negative effects for many of the procedures, there are hundreds of thousands of women and men who have cosmetic procedures with positive results. But as I tell my cosmetic acupuncture students during class, "If a procedure goes wrong on your face, you can't put a blouse over it."

COSMETIC ACUPUNCTURE

CHAPTER 10

Beauty is not who you are on the outside, it is
the wisdom and time you gave away to save
another struggling soul like you.

- Shannon L. Alder

NOW THAT I'VE covered some of the more dramatic options
with potential side effects for addressing visual aging, let
me introduce the healthiest alternative: Cosmetic Acupuncture,
also known as Facial Acupuncture. It is a unique anti-aging
treatment that not only enhances physical appearance but also
promotes overall health. In fact, Cosmetic Acupuncture is the
only anti-wrinkle, face-lifting procedure that enhances overall
health while delivering cosmetic results. Does a chemical peel
improve health? How about Botox® injections? Do they improve
your general health? No. The most effective way to achieve and
maintain a youthful appearance is to work from the inside out
or work on both the inside and the outside in ways that are
natural and safe.

In this chapter, we explore the history, benefits, and process
of Cosmetic Acupuncture, highlighting its effectiveness in real-
life case studies and providing a comprehensive understanding

of this time-honored technique. You'll discover how this holistic approach not only enhances your appearance but also promotes overall health and well-being.

Historical Background

Cosmetic Acupuncture is not new. Its roots dates back as early as the Sung Dynasty. Ancient Chinese texts, such as *The Nei Jing (The Yellow Emperor's Inner Classic)*, emphasized the connection between internal organ health and outward appearance. The results of treating the inside organ systems and channels show up on the outside: on your face, lips, and overall skin health. For centuries, various Chinese medical texts and practitioners have elaborated on these concepts, recommending food, herbs, and acupuncture for maintaining a youthful appearance. The technique that I developed and teach is called *Mei Zen Cosmetic Acupuncture,* and it has unique differences from other facial acupuncture techniques. Always ask your practitioner about the type of Cosmetic Acupuncture he or she practices, as well as the practitioner's training level because it is a sub-specialty of Chinese medicine.

Chinese medical books reflect the emphasis on using their medical system to maintain a youthful appearance. As far back as the Western Zhou period (1121–770 B.C.), Chinese practitioners made food recommendations to treat skin conditions. During the Warring States period (770–221 B.C.), the important text, *Shan Hai Jing (Classic of Mountains and Seas)*, described herbal remedies that were used for cosmetic purposes. This was followed by the *Shen Nong Ben Cao Jing (The Divine Husbandman's Classics of Materia Medica)*, an herbal material medica that included prescriptions for facial cosmetic results.

Later, acupuncture and herbal masks were added to texts. By the Song dynasty (960–1280 A.D.) the use of Chinese medicine for cosmetic purposes gained greater popularity. It was partly built upon the work of Sun Si Miao who, during the Tang dynasty (618–907 A.D.), developed many modalities that he said promoted health, longevity, and *beauty*. During the Ming dynasty (1368–1644 A.D.) Li Shi Shen, a highly esteemed physician, wrote *Ben Cao Gang Mu (Material Medica)*, a classic text that addresses specific parts of the face along with the complexion and wrinkles.

It's easy for me to be passionate about TCM and Cosmetic Acupuncture because it's a cosmetic procedure that is healthy, and I have seen its excellent results for over 20 years. Treating imbalances inside the body that cause aging and its effects in conjunction with treating the face and neck using acupuncture is simply, in my opinion, the best anti-aging medicine available. For example, I am the oldest of five, and all my younger siblings are fully gray, while I'm still barely salt and pepper. Why? Well, I've been using TCM for my health for 20+ years. First, preventing disease takes stress off the body. Also, I was the firstborn, so I received more of my parents' *Jing/Essence* than my siblings did. Receiving acupuncture treatments to balance my body, taking Chinese herbal prescriptions when needed, using Qigong as meditation, following TCM food guidelines, etc. have helped me age well. Preservation works!

Cosmetic Benefits of Cosmetic Acupuncture

When people receive modern cosmetic procedures, they don't care whether they improve their health—or whether it's healthy at all. When choosing Cosmetic Acupuncture, you get the best of both worlds. Along with improved overall health, there is the possibility of experiencing results from a natural treatment like Cosmetic Acupuncture. Here are just a few results from procedures that will help you look younger:

Reduction of Fine Lines

It's possible to reduce fine lines that may even disappear. Therefore, it is important to start Cosmetic Acupuncture in your 30s. It's a lot easier to prevent a wrinkle than it is to make it completely go away. Deeper lines may never go away completely, but they can soften and appear less harsh. And Cosmetic Acupuncture won't eliminate jowls or turkey neck, but it may define the jaw line in people whose necks are starting to sag.

Diminishing Acne and Rosacea

Cosmetic Acupuncture offers numerous benefits, including diminishing acne and rosacea, evening out overall skin tone by reducing redness, and fading age spots. It also improves facial muscle elasticity and boosts collagen production. As mentioned earlier, these improvements stem from the acupuncture needles creating tiny micro-traumas in the skin. When the skin perceives a trauma, fibroblasts rush to the site, producing collagen and elastin to heal the area. This natural wound-healing process restores and rejuvenates the skin, much like how your body repairs a cut, leaving the skin stronger and healthier.

Improved Skin Texture and Tone

Regular Cosmetic Acupuncture treatments can enhance your skin's texture and tone, making it appear smoother and more refined. This treatment stimulates blood flow and oxygenates the skin, which encourages cell regeneration and the removal of toxins. As new, healthier skin cells replace old ones, your skin develops a natural radiance and even tone. This process can also reduce the appearance of large pores, leaving the skin looking refreshed.

Boosted Facial Contour and Lift

Cosmetic Acupuncture can help promote a natural lift in areas that have started to lose elasticity, such as the cheeks, jawline, and brow. Unlike surgical options, which can appear dramatic or artificial, this treatment gently encourages the body's own collagen production, which subtly firms and lifts the skin. Over time, facial features may appear more defined, and sagging can become less noticeable, giving you a rejuvenated yet natural look.

Health Benefits of Cosmetic Acupuncture

Besides seeing "cosmetic" results, there are also general health results because Cosmetic Acupuncture treats the inside too! Here are some of the health effects I have seen in people who have had Cosmetic Acupuncture treatment:

- Feeling better as they receive the treatment
- Lessening of hot flashes and/or night sweats
- Balancing of internal body systems
- Increasing energy and becoming more invigorated
- Reducing mild depression and anxiety
- Improving digestion, which leads to better skin health

How Cosmetic Acupuncture Works from the Inside Out

According to the classical text *The Yellow Emperor's Inner Classic*, the energy from all the regular and extraordinary acupuncture channels meets at the neck and continues to the face and head. We find that treating acupuncture points on the body affects the face. The practitioner treats the overall body through acupuncture points before starting the cosmetic acupuncture procedure. It's a complete system of anti-aging.

According to Traditional Chinese Medicine (TCM), each organ system plays a role in controlling an aspect of beauty. The lungs influence the skin and body hair, as well as the skin's moisture. Balanced energy in the spleen and stomach affects the skin and lips, while the heart and small intestine manage the spirit, emotions, and digestion—reflected in the face. For instance, if emotional energy becomes unbalanced (linked to the heart and small intestine systems), anxiety and poor sleep can cause dark circles and puffiness under the eyes. Meanwhile, the kidney and bladder systems help maintain water balance and skin hydration. It makes perfect sense, then, that staying healthy and balanced internally is key to looking good externally.

The Procedure

Your practitioner will use pulse diagnosis to identify imbalances in your body. Pulse diagnosis is the premier method for making a diagnosis in Chinese medicine. The practitioner takes your pulses on both the left and right wrists, feeling the flow of energy through the channels (also known as meridians). During this part of the treatment, the practitioner decides which acupuncture points are needed. Your pulses are checked throughout the body treatment to ensure that your energy flows well. This diagnosis forms the basis of a personalized treatment plan tailored to address your individual health and cosmetic concerns. After the diagnosis and insertion of body acupuncture points, the facial or neck Cosmetic Acupuncture protocol will begin.

The Facial Needling

From the Chinese medicine perspective, putting acupuncture needles in the face or head causes oxygen and blood to rise to the face to lift the skin and improve the quality of the skin and fascia. From the modern medicine perspective, the insertion of acupuncture needles causes micro-traumas in the skin. The body perceives microtrauma as an injury and sends fibroblasts of collagen and elastin to the sites to heal the trauma. This response encourages collagen and elastin cells to grow in abundance. Unfortunately, as we age, our skin loses its capability to replace damaged collagen, so we need these procedures to boost collagen repair. Slowing collagen breakdown and increasing its supply is the only way to minimize wrinkling and sagging. The acupuncture needle is the perfect anti-aging tool!

The pattern of acupuncture points needled on the face retrains your skin to be more supple, elastic, and vibrant via its rejuvenating effect on your dermis that creates a lifting and smoothing effect. In the *Mei Zen* Cosmetic Acupuncture system, we use acupuncture points to give your skin its best opportunity for repair. Some facial acupuncture techniques target wrinkles, but *Mei Zen* practitioners use specific, prescribed acupuncture points.

For Acne Treatment

I treated a 25-year-old female with a lot of red acne scarring. Many times, we've been told that nothing will improve acne scarring although sometimes laser resurfacing or dermaplaning works, but there are no guarantees. Based on my experience, I was confident that Cosmetic Acupuncture would be effective in this case. How could it not? I knew it would rejuvenate and regulate her dermis, helping to reduce acne scarring and prevent future breakouts. I followed the protocol once a week.

Normally, after 40 years of age, it's a two times a week protocol, but for younger people, once a week may be sufficient. We saw results right away, so I continued the protocol once a week for 6 weeks, followed by every other week for another 4 treatments. There was a significant improvement in her skin! People were amazed because her skin became smooth, the redness disappeared, and there was barely any sign of scarring. It worked because we were healing the skin, not just putting something on it to cover up the redness and scarring. Her post-treatment includes monthly appointments or coming in pre-breakout. She also uses skin care products that nurture the skin rather than aggressively targeting acne.

Anti-Aging

In another case, I treated a 65-year-old woman with sagging eyelids, bagginess under the eyes, and quite a few lines on her cheeks. I performed the *Mei Zen* protocol two times a week for 5 weeks. Her eyelids raised and the bags below her eyes improved. In addition, the lines on her cheeks became less deep and her overall skin tone turned smooth with fewer age spots. Vertical lines on the cheeks can be a sign of unresolved grief, like tears, which requires emotional resolution to lessen the lines. Her maintenance requires appointments once a month. She also uses products to nourish skin, including special eye care products for the extra delicate skin around her eyes.

Sun Damage

I treated a 50-year-old woman who had extremely red cheeks from broken capillaries that occurred because of sun damage. It basically presents like tiny bruises under the skin that make the skin look really red. I applied the Mei Zen protocol 2 times a week for 5 weeks, and the broken capillaries healed, leaving her skin tone beautifully even. This is why everyone should wear sunscreen every day! She also sees me monthly for maintenance.

Sagging Chin Line

A female patient in her early 50s expressed she was worried about a sagging jawline. I talked with her about the importance of good digestion for keeping skin lifted and in good condition. For her, the neck protocol was appropriate because it includes acupuncture points on the face that affect the jawline and neck. After two treatments a week for five weeks, her jawline became more defined and the neck skin firmer. We have continued maintenance once a month, and she now uses all natural skin care products.

Is using Chinese medicine and a procedure like Cosmetic Acupuncture really the answer to our obsession with looking young? Well, it is a healthy cosmetic procedure compared to most other procedures. Because it is based on a system of preventive, healthy, energetic medicine, Cosmetic Acupuncture is excellent for your entire body and the treatments improve your overall health. The wrinkle reduction and vibrancy on your face is, in part, the result of overall improved health. The facial needling is also a healthy, relatively non-invasive way to improve the state of the skin. Cosmetic Acupuncture answers the looking-youthful obsession by improving or maintaining a youthful appearance and there's no potential for terrible side-effects like scarring or burning the skin.

Cosmetic Acupuncture stands out as a versatile and effective anti-aging treatment that promotes both physical appearance and overall health. By integrating ancient wisdom with modern techniques, it offers a comprehensive solution to the challenges of aging, ensuring a natural and lasting improvement in skin health and vitality.

CONCLUSION

CHAPTER 11

IN THIS BOOK, I wanted to share ideas and practices that we can use to "age victoriously." Basically, it's about the life choices we make and how to deal with the life we are living … that's it. I know that sounds trite. It's like someone saying, "Just deal with it." But that is kind of how it is. I'm not here to minimize your frustration with your body, the challenges you're facing in your family or job, or the weight of your losses. These experiences are real and deeply painful.

You might think it's been easy for me, but it hasn't. I've had injuries, symptoms, surgeries, failures … And my family's trauma has included a daughter with lupus who nearly died more than once, a very premature grandson in the NICU for 3 months, sudden death of loved ones, gigantic business losses. It's all caused worry, worry, worry and has required therapy. I feel especially fortunate to be a Chinese Medicine practitioner, with an entire system of medicine available to guide and support me through life with treatments and advice.

I had an interesting experience years ago, when one of my daughters required emergency surgery because of an injury. It wasn't life-threatening in the least, but more than two weeks later, I was still crying about it, ruminating about it … no, ruminating about her dying. That was my thought pattern. I'll never forget it. I was driving and wondering: what if she had died? Then I heard a loud booming voice say, "Even if she had died you would still be alive. You would have to live your life. You have family, friends, a life …" Who was talking to me? Some would say God. Some would say I was hallucinating. Some would say it was me. Doesn't matter. I got the message, and you should remember this message as well. You are still alive!

Maintaining good health is one of the most important factors in aging well. While this book highlights various ways to achieve this, it's helpful to take a step back and review the key practices. Here's a quick summary of the essential habits for promoting overall wellness and vitality.

Go back through the book and reflect on your answers to the questions. Have any of your answers or ideas changed, or do you have information to add to your responses after reading the book?

Are you following the advice outlined in the book? You can always go back to specific sections and follow the action steps outlined in each chapter.

Opinions about aging have evolved. While elders were once revered for their wisdom and experience, today, age is often met with resistance. Billions of dollars are poured into anti-aging therapies and procedures in pursuit of turning back the clock. But aging is a process—one that we can't stop, yet we do have some control over how we feel and navigate through it. As I said earlier in the book, "Time changes, our bodies change, and possibilities present themselves."

We've explored each decade of life, the changes that may arise, and strategies to help you feel and look your best. Nutrition plays a crucial role in preventing or minimizing age-related conditions. There are countless lifestyle choices that promote aging well—keeping your body moving, avoiding overeating, reducing alcohol intake, and giving up smoking are just a few that can have a tremendous impact on your overall well-being.

The clock keeps ticking, and nothing can stop it. But that doesn't mean you can't age gracefully, with intention, self-care, and plenty of self-love. You have a life to live, and how you choose to live it is up to you. My hope is that you take this journey with curiosity and joy. Discover the things that make you feel vibrant, fulfilled, and truly happy. Find what makes you feel alive and do it often—because aging well isn't just about looking good; it's about embracing every moment to live your fullest life.

REFERENCES

American Cancer Society.

Applied Psychology: Health and Well-Being, 3(1), 2011.

Arch Intern Med. (2012, June 11). 172(11), 837–844.

Ash, C. (n.d.). *Timeless Skin*.

Balch, P., & Balch, J. (n.d.). *Prescription for Nutritional Healing*.

BBC.co.uk.

Beauty Schools Directory. (n.d.). History of cosmetics.

Bensky, D., & Gamble, A. (n.d.). *Materia Medica*.

Bridges, L. (n.d.). *Face Reading in Chinese Medicine*.

CBS4Boston.com/team.

Chinatoday.com.

Chinese Charm. (n.d.). A brief history of beauty enhancement in China.

Colven, R. M., & Pinnell, S. R. (1996). Topical vitamin C in aging. *Clinics in Dermatology*, 14, 227–234.

Consumer Guide to Plastic Surgery.

CosmeticAcupunctureSeminars.com. (n.d.).

Danielsbacka, M. (2022). Grandparenting, health, and well-being: A systematic literature review. *European Journal of Aging*, 19, 341–368.

Deadman, P., Al-Khafaji, M., & Baker, K. (n.d.). *A Manual of Acupuncture*.

Du, C., et al. (2022). Relationships between dairy and calcium intake and mental health measures of higher education students in the U.S. *Nutrients*.

Ellinger, D., L.Ac. (n.d.). Clinical research and experience.

Finch, B. (n.d.). *Feng Shui and Chinese Astrology: Inside Chinese Metaphysics*.

Fitzpatrick, R. E., & Rostan, E. F. (2002). Double-blind, half-face study comparing topical vitamin C and vehicle for rejuvenation of photodamage. *Dermatologic Surgery*, 28, 231–236.

Free University Berlin. (n.d.). Research on the effects of stress on skin.

Hairhistory.com.

Humbert, P. G., et al. (2003). Topical ascorbic acid on photoaged skin: A double-blind study vs. placebo. *Experimental Dermatology*, 12, 237–244.

Int J Cardiol. (2013, April 15). 164(3), 267–276.

Johns, R. (n.d.). *The Art of Acupuncture Techniques*.

Johnson, J. A., Ph.D., D.M.Q. (n.d.). *Chinese Medical QiGong Therapy.*

Johnston, J. E., Psy.D. (n.d.). *Appearance Obsession.*

International Journal of Clinical Acupuncture. (1996).

Langer, E. J. (n.d.). *Counter Clockwise.*

Lavier, J., M.D. (n.d.). Article on Rejuvenessence.

Lee, M., O.M.D. (n.d.). *Master Tong's Acupuncture.*

Lin, J. Y., et al. (2003). UV photoprotection by combination topical antioxidants vitamin C and E. *Journal of the American Academy of Dermatology*, 48, 866–874.

Lucas, M., Ph.D., L.Ac. (n.d.). Clinical research and experience.

Mandolesi, L., et al. (2018). Effects of physical exercise on cognitive function and well-being. *Frontiers in Psychology.*

Manosso, L. M., et al. (2020). Vitamin E for managing major depressive disorder. *Nutrition Neuroscience.*

Ni, M., Ph.D., & McNease, C. (n.d.). *The Tao of Nutrition.*

Maciocia, G. (n.d.). *Diagnosis in Chinese Medicine: A Comprehensive Guide.*

Mariet, E. (n.d.). *Essentials of Human Anatomy and Physiology.*

Medicinenet.com.

Nutrients. (2011, April). 3(4), 385–428.

Office of Dietary Supplements, NIH.

Ohashi, with Moore, T. (n.d.). *Reading the Body: Ohashi's Book of Oriental Diagnosis.*

Ojeda, L., Ph.D. (n.d.). *Menopause without Medicine.*

Perez, C. C. (n.d.). *Invisible Women: Data Bias in a World Designed for Men.*

Perricone, N., M.D. (n.d.). *The Wrinkle Cure.*

Phillips, C. L., Combs, S. B., & Pinnell, S. R. (1994). Effects of ascorbic acid on collagen synthesis. *Journal of Investigative Dermatology*, 103, 228–232.

Pitchford, P. (n.d.). *Healing with Whole Foods.*

Plasticsurgery.org.

Positivehealth.com.

Postgrad Med J. (1979, June). 55(644), 373–376.

Prasad, K. N., Ph.D., & Prasad, M.D., K. C. (n.d.). *Fight Cancer with Vitamins and Supplements.*

Prevention Magazine. (2008, June).

Proc Natl Acad Sci USA. (2011, Nov 8). 108(45), 18244–18248.

Ramholz, J., O.M.D. (n.d.). Teacher, mentor.

Rosen, R., O.M.D. (n.d.). Teacher.

Shanghai College of Traditional Medicine. (n.d.). *Acupuncture: A Comprehensive Text*.

Swerdlow, J. L. (2002, November). Unmasking skin. *National Geographic*.

Thermage.com.

Tourles, S. (n.d.). *Naturally Healthy Skin: Techniques for a Lifetime of Radiant Skin*.

UNC Fertility Center.

Walter, N., et al. (2019). Effects of self-talk training on athletes. *Sports*.

WebMD.com.

Yao, Z. G. (n.d.). Master; Medical QiGong internship (Lucas).

Yin, G. (n.d.). *Three Needle Technique*.

Lucas, M., Ph.D., L.Ac., & Ellinger, D., L.Ac. (n.d.). *You Don't Need Botox®: Defy Aging the Natural, Healthy Way*.

Zhu, M. (n.d.). *Zhu's Scalp Acupuncture*.

Also by Dr. Martha Lucas

Catholic Daughters of Catholic Mothers:
A Memoir & Guided Journal

52 Weeks of Victorious Aging:
Tips to Ensure a Happy and Healthy Year at Any Age

Pulse Diagnosis: Beyond Slippery and Wiry:
Key to the Practice of TCM!

Cosmetic Acupuncture Works!:
Your Guide to Cosmetic Acupuncture for Anti-Aging

ABOUT THE AUTHOR

Dr. Martha Lucas, L.Ac., is a leading expert in holistic health, holding a Ph.D. in Psychology and extensive experience as a Practitioner of Chinese Medicine. Passionate about natural approaches to wellness, Dr. Lucas has dedicated years to researching and practicing techniques that promote longevity, vitality, and graceful aging—without relying on invasive procedures or synthetic solutions.

In her latest book on natural anti-aging, she combines the wisdom of Eastern medicine with modern psychological insights to help readers unlock their body's innate ability to heal and rejuvenate.

Ready to take control of your health and embrace a vibrant, youthful life? Dive into the book today and begin your journey toward natural, lasting wellness!

More Info

acupuncturewoman.com
lucasteachings.com
myzenskincare.com

ABOUT THE PUBLISHER

ArmLin House is a unique publisher and production company. We help you develop your story in a memoir, business book, instructional video, and more. Then we format your story and help you present your work, whether you release it yourself or we do it for you. And once your story is out there, we can help you promote it with written and visual aids.

It's our mission to help our clients succeed in whatever they do. We take your visions and make them possible through coaching and distribution assistance. The products we help produce are informational and entertaining, as well as help you market yourself and your business. We produce based on your needs, whether it be in print, digital, audio, or video formats. Then we help release it to a worldwide audience.

More Info

armlinhouse.com

52 WEEKS OF VICTORIOUS AGING
TIPS TO ENSURE A HAPPY AND HEALTHY YEAR AT ANY AGE

Enjoy The Companion to This Book!

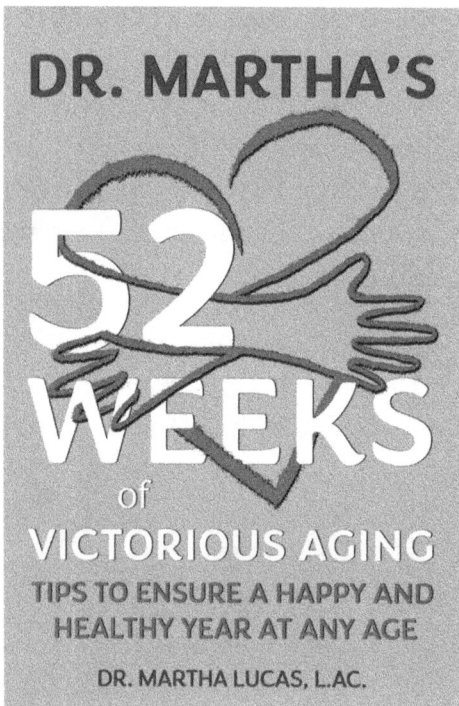

Create a healthier, happier you as you advance in years. It's Victorious Aging!

Dr. Martha provides 52 health and happiness actions that you can realistically incorporate into your life. Each tip is designed to create a healthier you as you advance in years. No one is too young to start. And you only have to accomplish one tip a week.

You Can Start Any Day or Week in the Year.

Beautifully illustrated, this book pairs weekly tips with engaging visuals that inspire reflection and make the journey toward Victorious Aging both practical and enjoyable.

A GREAT GIFT!

family weekends sunny days

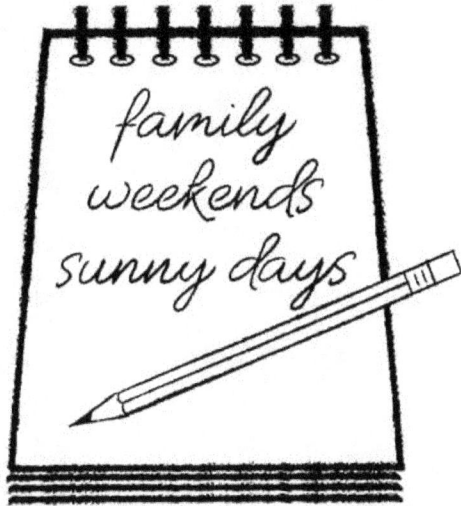

There are no dates in this book. Most of us don't need another complicated thing to do each day, let alone try to remember to read every day. Once a week is perfect! You choose. Set an alarm or reminder to start the week, read a tip midweek, or end your week on a high note with a weekly tip.

"I have this book on my Kindle so that I can read a weekly tip and strive to reach that mindset or goal. And I often refer to the tip throughout the week. It's a great little bible of useful information for me."

Dr. Martha Lucas loves working with patients in her office, online, and through her books. Buy Dr. Martha's 52 Weeks of Victorious Aging: Tips to Ensure a Happy and Healthy Year at Any Age and she'll help you start improving your quality of life NOW!

www.ingramcontent.com/pod-product-compliance
Lightning Source LLC
Chambersburg PA
CBHW060227030426
42335CB00014B/1357